The Complete Guide to Quiet BPD

Evidence-Based Strategies for Managing High-Functioning Borderline Personality Disorder

Paul Fabunni Meredith

ISBN: 978-1-7642471-2-2

Table of Contents

Chapter 1: When borderline turns inward

Holly sat in yet another therapist's office, watching Dr. Martinez's face shift from professional concern to something that looked suspiciously like relief. "I think we've done all we can together," he said, his words carrying the familiar sting of rejection wrapped in clinical language. Three therapists had terminated her treatment in two years. Three professionals had essentially told her she was too much—or perhaps, paradoxically, not enough—for their expertise. The irony wasn't lost on Holly: she appeared so composed, so functional, that even mental health professionals couldn't see her drowning beneath the surface.

This story repeats itself countless times across therapy offices worldwide. People with quiet borderline personality disorder (BPD) face a unique challenge—their pain is invisible, their struggles dismissed, their very real mental health condition overlooked because it doesn't match the dramatic presentation most people associate with BPD. You might be reading this because you recognize yourself in Holly's experience, or perhaps you're trying to understand someone you care about who seems fine on the outside but battles tremendous internal storms.

The hidden face of emotional turmoil

Quiet BPD represents what clinicians call the "discouraged" subtype of borderline personality disorder—a presentation that turns all the classic symptoms inward rather than outward. Instead of explosive arguments or dramatic gestures, individuals with quiet BPD engage in silent self-punishment, internal emotional chaos, and a relentless pursuit of perfection that masks deep-seated fears of abandonment and rejection.

The diagnostic criteria for BPD remain the same across all presentations, but quiet BPD manifests these symptoms in ways that often fly under the radar. You won't find dramatic suicide threats or volatile relationships that make headlines. Instead, you'll discover people who:

- Maintain stable careers while battling crippling self-doubt
- Keep long-term relationships while secretly fearing abandonment
- Appear calm and collected while experiencing emotional hurricanes internally
- Excel academically or professionally while struggling with persistent feelings of emptiness

Dr. Sarah Chen, who has specialized in quiet BPD for over fifteen years, explains that these individuals often present as the "model patient" in therapy—articulate, insightful, and seemingly motivated. Yet this same presentation can lead to misdiagnosis or treatment that doesn't address the underlying borderline dynamics.

What makes quiet BPD different from classic presentations

The distinction between quiet BPD and classic BPD isn't about severity—both cause significant distress and impairment. The difference lies in expression. Classic BPD tends to be externally focused: relationships become battlegrounds, emotions explode outward, and the struggle is visible to others. Quiet BPD turns inward: relationships become sources of secret anxiety, emotions implode rather than explode, and the struggle remains largely invisible.

Consider Maria, a 28-year-old software engineer who maintains excellent work performance reviews while secretly checking her phone dozens of times daily, analyzing every text message from friends for signs of rejection. Her classic BPD counterpart might bombard friends with calls or show up unannounced at their homes. Maria simply withdraws when she feels threatened, punishing herself with harsh internal criticism and social isolation.

The emotional dysregulation remains the same—intense, rapid mood shifts that feel overwhelming and uncontrollable. However, quiet BPD individuals have learned to contain these emotional storms, often at significant psychological cost. They might experience the same level of emotional pain as someone with classic BPD but express it through:

2

- Self-harm that leaves no visible marks
- Eating disorders or other hidden self-destructive behaviors
- Perfectionism that becomes self-punishment
- Social withdrawal instead of dramatic confrontations
- Internal self-criticism rather than external blame

The four faces of quiet BPD

Research and clinical observation reveal four primary presentations within quiet BPD, though individuals often display characteristics from multiple categories:

The Perfectionist operates under the belief that flawless performance will prevent abandonment or criticism. Sarah, a 35-year-old marketing director, spends hours rewriting emails to colleagues, missing deadlines because nothing feels good enough to send. She's received promotions and praise throughout her career, yet lives in constant fear that people will discover she's "fraudulent." Her perfectionism isn't about achievement—it's armor against the terrifying possibility of rejection.

The People-Pleaser sacrifices personal needs and boundaries to maintain relationships and avoid conflict. James, a 31-year-old teacher, says yes to every social invitation, volunteer opportunity, and extra work assignment, even when exhausted. He's developed chronic fatigue and anxiety from constantly monitoring others' moods and adjusting his behavior accordingly. His people-pleasing stems from the deep-seated belief that his authentic self is unlovable and that others will abandon him if he ever says no or expresses disagreement.

The Self-Punisher directs all anger and frustration inward, engaging in various forms of self-harm or self-sabotage. Rebecca, a 29-year-old nurse, maintains excellent professional relationships and is considered reliable by colleagues and friends. However, when she perceives rejection or makes mistakes, she engages in covert self-harm— scratching until she bleeds, restricting food intake, or deliberately isolating herself during times when she most needs support. Her self-punishment feels like justice for being "defective" or "too much."

The Avoider withdraws from relationships and opportunities to prevent potential rejection or abandonment. Michael, a 33-year-old graphic designer, has exceptional creative talent but works freelance from home to avoid office politics and interpersonal complications. He's turned down job offers, declined dates, and maintains surface-level friendships to protect himself from the vulnerability that deeper connections require. His avoidance provides immediate relief from social anxiety but reinforces his belief that he's fundamentally unfit for meaningful relationships.

Clinical understanding within diagnostic frameworks

The current Diagnostic and Statistical Manual (DSM-5) doesn't specifically categorize quiet BPD as a separate diagnosis but recognizes it within the broader BPD criteria. The nine diagnostic criteria for BPD include:

1. Frantic efforts to avoid real or imagined abandonment
2. Unstable and intense interpersonal relationships
3. Identity disturbance and unstable self-image
4. Impulsivity in potentially damaging areas
5. Recurrent suicidal behavior or self-mutilating behavior
6. Emotional instability due to mood reactivity
7. Chronic feelings of emptiness
8. Inappropriate intense anger or difficulty controlling anger
9. Transient stress-related paranoid ideation or severe dissociative symptoms

In quiet BPD, these criteria manifest internally rather than externally. The abandonment fears remain intense but lead to withdrawal rather than clinging behaviors. Relationships feel unstable internally even when they appear stable to observers. Identity disturbance occurs through chronic self-doubt and shape-shifting to please others rather than dramatic identity shifts. Impulsivity might manifest as workaholism, perfectionism, or secret self-destructive behaviors rather than obvious risk-taking.

4

Neuroscientifically, individuals with quiet BPD show the same amygdala hyperactivity and prefrontal cortex dysfunction found in classic BPD. However, they've developed stronger inhibitory mechanisms—often through childhood experiences that punished emotional expression. This creates a pattern where emotional intensity remains high, but expression becomes suppressed, leading to internal rather than external chaos.

Recognizing quiet BPD in yourself

If you suspect you might have quiet BPD, consider these patterns in your daily experience:

Emotional experiences: Do you feel emotions intensely but struggle to express them? Do small interactions replay in your mind for hours or days? Do you experience sudden mood shifts that others don't notice but feel overwhelming to you?

Relationship patterns: Do you analyze conversations obsessively for signs of rejection? Do you withdraw when feeling hurt rather than addressing issues directly? Do you maintain relationships by constantly adapting yourself to what you think others want?

Self-perception: Do you feel like you're wearing a mask most of the time? Do you struggle with persistent feelings that you're somehow defective or too much for others? Do you have difficulty knowing what you actually want or need?

Coping mechanisms: Do you use perfectionism, people-pleasing, or achievement to feel worthy? Do you engage in hidden self-destructive behaviors when feeling overwhelmed? Do you isolate yourself when stressed rather than seeking support?

Daily functioning: Do you appear highly functional to others while feeling barely able to manage internally? Do you exhaust yourself maintaining your composed exterior? Do you feel like you're constantly performing rather than living authentically?

The journey toward recognition and healing

Holly's story didn't end with that third therapist's termination. She eventually found Dr. Patricia Williams, a clinician trained specifically in quiet BPD presentations. Dr. Williams recognized the signs that previous therapists had missed: the over-apologizing, the hyper-responsibility for others' emotions, the careful monitoring of her own expressions and tone. More importantly, she understood that Holly's composed exterior masked the same emotional dysregulation found in more obvious BPD presentations.

Recognition represents the first step toward healing. For many people with quiet BPD, simply understanding that their internal experience has a name and that effective treatments exist brings tremendous relief. You're not "too sensitive" or "just anxious"—you're dealing with a recognized mental health condition that responds well to appropriate treatment.

The path forward involves learning to express emotions safely, developing authentic relationships, and building a sense of self that doesn't depend on others' approval. This work requires patience, as quiet BPD often develops over many years of learning to suppress emotional needs. However, with proper understanding and support, people with quiet BPD can develop the emotional skills needed for authentic, fulfilling relationships and a genuine sense of self-worth.

Understanding quiet BPD also requires recognizing its strengths. Many individuals with this condition possess exceptional empathy, creativity, and emotional intelligence. They often excel in caregiving professions and bring deep sensitivity to their relationships and work. The goal isn't to eliminate these qualities but to help them exist without the accompanying self-judgment and internal turmoil.

Key insights for understanding

Essential points to remember:

- Quiet BPD represents an internalized version of borderline personality disorder where symptoms turn inward rather than outward
- The four main presentations include perfectionist, people-pleaser, self-punisher, and avoider patterns, often overlapping in individuals
- Diagnostic criteria remain the same as classic BPD, but manifestations appear as internal emotional chaos rather than external drama
- Recognition and proper diagnosis often take longer due to the hidden nature of symptoms and tendency for misdiagnosis
- Treatment approaches must account for the unique presentation while addressing underlying emotional dysregulation
- Individuals with quiet BPD often possess significant strengths including empathy, emotional intelligence, and creative abilities that can support their healing journey

The next chapter will examine how this internalized struggle creates the paradox of appearing highly functional while experiencing significant internal distress—a phenomenon that confuses both individuals and their support systems.

Chapter 2: Behind the high-functioning facade

Dr. Amanda Richardson appears to have everything figured out. At 32, she's completed her residency at Harvard Medical School, maintains an impressive research publication record, and colleagues consistently describe her as composed, insightful, and reliable. Her apartment showcases tasteful art, her social media reflects carefully curated success, and her professional trajectory suggests someone who has mastered both medicine and life. Yet Amanda spends most evenings curled in her bathroom floor, sobbing uncontrollably while simultaneously berating herself for being "too emotional" and "not grateful enough" for her achievements.

This jarring contrast between external success and internal torment defines the daily reality for many people with quiet BPD. You might recognize this pattern in your own life—others see competence and achievement while you experience constant internal storms, self-doubt, and emotional exhaustion. This chapter explores the complex dynamics behind high-functioning quiet BPD and helps explain why appearing "fine" can actually complicate recognition and treatment of this condition.

The perfectionist's paradox

Amanda's story illustrates what clinicians call the "high-functioning" presentation of quiet BPD, where individuals achieve external success while battling internal chaos. Her achievements aren't coincidental to her BPD—they're often direct results of it. The same emotional intensity that causes internal suffering also fuels exceptional performance, attention to detail, and sensitivity to others' needs that can translate into professional success.

Consider Amanda's typical workday: she arrives at the hospital an hour early to review patient files, not because she's unprepared but because she's terrified of making mistakes that might reveal her perceived incompetence. During medical rounds, she carefully monitors attending physicians' facial expressions, adjusting her contributions based on subtle cues others might miss entirely. Her comprehensive patient notes earn praise from supervisors, though she rewrites them multiple times because nothing feels adequate. Colleagues see dedication and thoroughness; Amanda experiences relentless anxiety and exhaustion.

The emotional dysregulation that characterizes BPD manifests differently in high-functioning presentations. Instead of dramatic outbursts, emotions get channeled into achievement, perfectionism, and hyper-responsibility. Amanda's emotional intensity becomes fuel for 80-hour work weeks, meticulous attention to detail, and an uncanny ability to anticipate problems before they occur. These skills make her valuable to employers and admired by peers, yet they stem from the same neurobiological differences that cause her bathroom floor breakdowns.

Dr. Michael Torres, who researches high-functioning BPD at Stanford University, explains that these individuals often develop what he calls "compensatory excellence"—using achievement and external validation to manage internal emotional chaos. The strategy works partially, providing temporary relief from feelings of emptiness and inadequacy, but ultimately becomes exhausting and unsustainable.

Neurobiological differences that whisper instead of scream

Brain imaging studies reveal that individuals with quiet BPD show the same neurobiological patterns as those with classic BPD—hyperactive amygdala responses to perceived threats and reduced prefrontal cortex regulation of emotional responses. However, quiet BPD individuals have typically developed stronger inhibitory mechanisms, often learned during childhood experiences that punished emotional expression.

Amanda's brain shows typical BPD patterns: her amygdala fires intensely when she perceives potential criticism or rejection, flooding her system with stress hormones. However, her prefrontal cortex has learned to suppress external expression of these emotions through

9

years of practice. This creates a situation where emotional intensity remains high, but behavioral expression gets contained, leading to internal rather than external chaos.

The neurobiological reality explains why Amanda can perform complex medical procedures while experiencing emotional turmoil. Her cognitive abilities remain intact even during emotional storms because the parts of her brain responsible for technical skills continue functioning normally. However, the emotional regulation systems remain dysregulated, creating the jarring contrast between professional competence and personal distress.

Dr. Sarah Kim's research at UCLA demonstrates that high-functioning BPD individuals often show enhanced activity in brain regions associated with self-monitoring and behavioral inhibition. This enhanced self-control allows them to maintain professional performance but comes at significant metabolic cost—their brains work overtime to maintain composure, leading to chronic fatigue and emotional exhaustion.

Gender differences in presentation and recognition

Research consistently shows that women receive BPD diagnoses more frequently than men, with estimates ranging from 65% to 85% of diagnoses being female. However, this disparity likely reflects diagnostic bias rather than actual prevalence differences. Men with quiet BPD often receive alternative diagnoses or go unrecognized entirely because their presentations don't match stereotypical BPD presentations.

Marcus, a 38-year-old investment banker, exemplifies male quiet BPD. His emotional storms manifest as workaholism, sexual compulsivity, and substance use rather than the self-harm or eating disorders more commonly associated with female presentations. He maintains excellent professional relationships while secretly struggling with persistent emptiness and fears of abandonment. His masculine socialization taught him that emotional expression equals weakness, so his BPD symptoms get channeled into socially acceptable male behaviors like excessive work, exercise, or sexual conquest.

Female presentations of quiet BPD often involve perfectionism, people-pleasing, and eating disorders—behaviors that align with feminine social expectations and may be dismissed as "normal" female concerns. Amanda's drive for perfection and her tendency to prioritize others' needs might be seen as admirable feminine qualities rather than symptoms of emotional dysregulation requiring treatment.

These gender differences create significant diagnostic challenges. Mental health professionals trained to recognize classic BPD presentations might miss quiet BPD entirely, particularly in male patients whose symptoms don't match expected patterns. This contributes to prolonged suffering and inappropriate treatment approaches that don't address underlying emotional dysregulation.

Cultural factors that shape symptom expression

Cultural background significantly influences how quiet BPD symptoms manifest and how individuals cope with emotional dysregulation. Collectivist cultures that emphasize group harmony and emotional restraint may actually promote quiet BPD presentations by discouraging direct emotional expression and encouraging self-sacrifice for family or community good.

Kenji, a 29-year-old second-generation Japanese-American software developer, illustrates these cultural dynamics. His family's emphasis on emotional restraint, academic achievement, and bringing honor to the family name shaped his quiet BPD presentation. His emotional storms get channeled into perfectionist work performance and an overwhelming sense of responsibility for his parents' happiness and pride. His cultural background makes his symptoms appear virtuous rather than pathological, delaying recognition and treatment.

Similarly, cultural attitudes toward mental health affect help-seeking behaviors. In cultures that stigmatize mental health treatment or view emotional struggles as personal weaknesses, individuals with quiet

BPD may resist seeking help or may present their concerns in ways that obscure the underlying emotional dysregulation. They might focus on physical symptoms, work stress, or relationship concerns rather than acknowledging the emotional chaos that underlies these surface issues.

Religious and spiritual backgrounds can both help and hinder recognition of quiet BPD. Some individuals find that meditation, prayer, or spiritual community provides emotional regulation skills that help manage BPD symptoms. However, religious emphasis on self-sacrifice, humility, and emotional restraint might also reinforce quiet BPD patterns by framing self-punishment and people-pleasing as spiritual virtues rather than symptoms requiring attention.

Why clinicians miss the diagnosis

Mental health professionals face unique challenges when working with high-functioning quiet BPD clients. These individuals often present as ideal patients—articulate, insightful, motivated, and compliant with treatment recommendations. They rarely miss appointments, complete homework assignments thoroughly, and provide detailed accounts of their emotional experiences. This presentation can actually work against accurate diagnosis and effective treatment.

Dr. Jennifer Martinez, a clinical psychologist with twenty years of experience, describes her initial encounters with quiet BPD clients: "They seemed to have such good insight into their patterns and such strong motivation to change that I assumed traditional cognitive-behavioral approaches would work quickly. It took months to recognize that their apparent insight was actually intellectualization—a way of staying in their heads to avoid feeling emotions that felt dangerous."

The absence of dramatic presentations that typically prompt BPD diagnosis means that quiet BPD individuals often receive diagnoses like generalized anxiety disorder, major depression, or adjustment disorders. These diagnoses aren't necessarily wrong—many people with quiet BPD do experience anxiety and depression—but they miss the underlying emotional dysregulation that drives these symptoms.

Additionally, quiet BPD individuals often possess exceptional emotional intelligence and interpersonal skills that can mask their struggles. They're adept at reading others' emotions, anticipating needs, and adjusting their behavior accordingly. These skills can make them appear psychologically healthy and interpersonally mature, obscuring the internal chaos and identity disturbance that characterizes their actual experience.

The therapeutic relationship itself can become complicated with quiet BPD clients. Their sensitivity to perceived criticism or rejection might lead them to carefully monitor their therapist's responses and adjust their presentations accordingly. They might become the "perfect client," sharing insights they think their therapist wants to hear while carefully avoiding topics that feel too vulnerable or potentially rejecting.

The exhaustion of constant performance

Perhaps the most defining characteristic of high-functioning quiet BPD is the tremendous energy required to maintain external composure while managing internal emotional storms. Amanda describes her daily experience as "wearing a full-body costume that never comes off"—every social interaction requires conscious effort to monitor her expressions, tone, and responses to ensure others don't detect her internal struggles.

This constant performance creates several interconnected problems:

Emotional exhaustion: Suppressing natural emotional responses requires significant mental energy. By evening, Amanda feels drained not from medical procedures but from managing her internal emotional state while appearing competent and composed to others.

Identity confusion: Spending so much energy on external presentation makes it difficult to know what authentic thoughts and

13

feelings actually are. Amanda sometimes lies awake wondering if her professional interests are genuine or just another performance designed to gain approval.

Relationship difficulties: Maintaining facades in relationships prevents genuine intimacy. Amanda's friends see her as stable and supportive but rarely get to see her vulnerabilities or genuine emotional needs, creating relationships that feel one-sided and ultimately unsatisfying.

Burnout cycles: The combination of perfectionist work habits and emotional suppression often leads to periodic burnouts where maintaining the facade becomes temporarily impossible. Amanda experiences these as mysterious episodes where she can barely function, feeling guilty for being "weak" without understanding the underlying emotional dynamics.

The hidden strengths within the struggle

High-functioning quiet BPD isn't simply a matter of better coping skills—it often reflects genuine strengths that develop alongside emotional dysregulation. Amanda's emotional sensitivity, while sometimes overwhelming, also makes her an exceptional physician. She notices subtle changes in patients' conditions, picks up on family dynamics that affect treatment adherence, and provides compassionate care that colleagues and patients consistently value.

The perfectionist tendencies that cause Amanda personal distress also contribute to medical outcomes. Her meticulous attention to detail prevents errors, her thorough documentation helps other healthcare providers, and her drive to continuously improve her skills makes her an asset to her medical team. These qualities aren't separate from her BPD—they're often direct expressions of the same emotional intensity and interpersonal sensitivity that characterize the condition.

Many high-functioning individuals with quiet BPD possess exceptional creative abilities, empathetic understanding, and innovative problem-solving skills. Their emotional intensity, when channeled productively, can fuel artistic expression, compassionate caregiving, and breakthrough insights in various fields. The goal of treatment isn't to eliminate these qualities but to help them exist without the accompanying self-judgment and internal suffering.

Breaking through the facade

Recognition and treatment of high-functioning quiet BPD requires looking beyond external achievements to understand internal experiences. Amanda's breakthrough came not through listing her symptoms but through recognizing the tremendous effort required to maintain her composed exterior and the emotional exhaustion that resulted.

Effective treatment for high-functioning quiet BPD must address both the underlying emotional dysregulation and the perfectionist patterns that mask it. This often means learning to tolerate imperfection, express authentic emotions safely, and develop relationships that don't require constant performance.

The journey involves recognizing that high functioning might actually be a sophisticated form of emotional avoidance rather than genuine psychological health. True recovery means being able to experience and express emotions authentically while maintaining the genuine strengths and abilities that high-functioning individuals possess.

Essential insights

Key points for understanding high-functioning quiet BPD:

- External success and achievement can mask significant internal emotional dysregulation and distress
- Perfectionism and people-pleasing often represent attempts to manage underlying fears of abandonment and rejection
- Gender and cultural factors significantly influence how quiet BPD symptoms are expressed and recognized

15

- Mental health professionals may miss the diagnosis due to the absence of dramatic presentations typically associated with BPD
- The constant effort required to maintain composure while managing internal storms leads to chronic exhaustion and burnout
- High-functioning individuals with quiet BPD often possess genuine strengths including empathy, creativity, and emotional intelligence
- Effective treatment must address underlying emotional dysregulation while honoring the real abilities and qualities that individuals have developed

The next chapter will explore how quiet BPD develops, examining the complex interplay between genetics, temperament, and environmental factors that create the perfect storm for internalized emotional dysregulation.

Chapter 3: The perfect storm: Origins and development

Rachel's childhood appeared idyllic from the outside—sprawling suburban home, involved parents who attended every school event, academic achievements that earned family pride, and a social circle that seemed supportive and stable. Her parents, both successful professionals, provided material comfort and maintained the family's reputation as pillars of their community. Yet beneath this polished exterior, Rachel learned early that her emotional needs were inconvenient disruptions to family harmony, that sensitivity was weakness, and that love was earned through achievement rather than given unconditionally.

Today, Rachel advocates publicly for mental health awareness and speaks openly about her journey with quiet BPD. Her transformation from emotionally suppressed high achiever to authentic advocate illustrates how understanding the origins of quiet BPD can illuminate pathways toward healing. This chapter examines the complex interplay of factors that create the conditions for quiet BPD to develop, helping you understand how seemingly normal childhood experiences can contribute to significant adult emotional dysregulation.

The invisible wounds of emotional neglect

Dr. Jonice Webb's groundbreaking research on childhood emotional neglect reveals how children can experience profound emotional wounds even in families that appear loving and functional. Unlike physical abuse or dramatic trauma, emotional neglect occurs through omission rather than commission—what doesn't happen rather than what does happen. For many people with quiet BPD, this subtle form of childhood adversity proves far more influential than obvious trauma in shaping their adult emotional patterns.

Rachel's parents weren't cruel or intentionally harmful. Her father, a successful attorney, worked long hours to provide for the family and showed love through financial provision and involvement in Rachel's academic achievements. Her mother, a part-time nurse who returned to work when Rachel started school, demonstrated care through perfectly prepared meals, clean clothes, and organized schedules. Neither parent possessed emotional awareness or regulation skills themselves, having grown up in similar emotionally restrained environments.

The emotional neglect in Rachel's childhood manifested in subtle but profound ways:

Dismissal of emotions: When Rachel felt scared after a nightmare, her parents would quickly reassure her that "everything's fine" without acknowledging or helping her process the fear itself. When she felt excited about friendships or interests, her enthusiasm was met with gentle reminders to "calm down" or "not get too carried away."

Achievement-based worth: Rachel learned that her value to her parents correlated directly with her accomplishments. Good grades, athletic achievements, and social success earned attention and praise, while struggles or failures resulted in disappointed silence or suggestions for improvement.

Emotional perfectionism: The family's unspoken rule was that negative emotions were problems to be solved quickly rather than experiences to be understood and processed. Rachel learned to suppress sadness, anger, and fear because expressing these emotions created discomfort in her parents and disrupted family peace.

Covert invalidation: Rachel's parents didn't directly tell her that her emotions were wrong, but their responses consistently communicated that emotional experiences were less important than maintaining composure and achieving goals.

This pattern of emotional neglect teaches children that their internal emotional world is somehow defective or inappropriate. They learn to disconnect from their own emotional experiences while becoming hyper-attuned to others' emotional needs and expectations. This creates the foundation for quiet BPD: intense emotions that feel dangerous to express, identity confusion about what constitutes authentic self-expression, and relationship patterns based on performance rather than genuine connection.

The highly sensitive child who learned to hide

Temperament research demonstrates that some children are born with heightened emotional sensitivity—they feel emotions more intensely, react more strongly to environmental stimuli, and require more support to regulate emotional responses. Dr. Elaine Aron's research on highly sensitive persons reveals that approximately 20% of people possess this trait, which can become either a profound strength or source of significant distress depending on how others respond to it.

Rachel displayed classic signs of high sensitivity from early childhood. She felt overwhelmed by loud noises, bright lights, and chaotic environments. She noticed subtle changes in others' moods and often became distressed when sensing tension between her parents or teachers. She formed intense attachments to friends and felt devastated when relationships shifted or ended. Her emotional responses to movies, books, and real-life events were more intense than her peers', leading to teasing and social difficulties.

In emotionally supportive families, highly sensitive children learn that their emotional intensity is a gift that can be channeled productively. They receive help developing emotional regulation skills and learn to see their sensitivity as empathy and emotional intelligence. However, in families that lack emotional awareness or view sensitivity as problematic, these children learn to suppress their natural emotional responses and develop shame about their temperamental traits.

Rachel's parents, both raised in emotionally restrictive environments themselves, didn't understand how to support a highly sensitive child. They interpreted her emotional reactions as "overreacting" and consistently encouraged her to be "more like other kids" who seemed less affected by emotional stimuli. This well-meaning but misguided response taught Rachel that her natural temperament was somehow defective and needed correction.

The combination of high sensitivity and emotional invalidation creates ideal conditions for quiet BPD development. The child possesses intense emotions that feel overwhelming and unmanageable, but learns that expressing these emotions results in rejection or criticism. They develop sophisticated strategies for suppressing emotional expression while the underlying emotional intensity continues unabated.

Intergenerational transmission of emotional suppression

Mental health conditions often run in families, but the transmission isn't simply genetic. Emotional regulation skills, relationship patterns, and attitudes toward feelings get passed down through generations, creating family systems where emotional suppression becomes normalized and even valued.

Rachel's father grew up in a military family where emotional restraint was considered strength and emotional expression was viewed as weakness. His father, a career officer, taught him that successful men control their emotions and focus on achievement and duty. Rachel's father learned these lessons well, becoming a successful professional who prided himself on remaining calm under pressure and making logical rather than emotional decisions.

Rachel's mother's family emphasized social harmony and avoiding conflict at all costs. Her mother learned to suppress any emotions that might disturb family peace and to take responsibility for managing others' emotional states. She became exceptionally skilled at reading social cues and adjusting her behavior to maintain relationships, but never learned to identify or express her own authentic emotional needs.

Both parents unconsciously recreated their childhood emotional environments in their own family. They didn't intend to emotionally neglect Rachel—they were providing the same type of care they had received and that they believed had made them successful adults. However, their lack of emotional awareness and regulation skills meant they couldn't teach Rachel what they had never learned themselves.

This intergenerational pattern explains why quiet BPD often occurs in families that appear loving and functional. The emotional neglect isn't intentional or malicious—it's simply the continuation of patterns that have been passed down through generations of well-meaning parents who lacked emotional awareness and skills.

Dr. Patricia Steele's research on family systems and BPD demonstrates that parents don't need to be abusive or obviously dysfunctional to contribute to BPD development in their children. Sometimes loving parents who struggle with their own emotional regulation inadvertently create environments where children learn that emotions are dangerous and that love must be earned through performance rather than received unconditionally.

When trauma wears expensive clothes

Not all quiet BPD develops in overtly neglectful environments. Sometimes trauma occurs within families that possess significant resources, education, and social status—contexts where the emotional wounds are particularly difficult to recognize and address because they contradict external appearances of success and stability.

Consider Alexandra's story: daughter of two physicians, raised in an affluent suburb with every material advantage. Her parents' demanding careers meant long hours and high stress levels that they brought home regularly. Family dinners involved discussions of medical cases, academic expectations, and social obligations rather than emotional connection or personal sharing. Alexandra learned that her worth came through academic achievement and that emotional needs were selfish distractions from more important goals.

The trauma in Alexandra's childhood wasn't physical abuse or neglect in traditional senses. Instead, it was the trauma of having to suppress her authentic self to meet family expectations, of learning that love was conditional on performance, and of developing an identity based entirely on others' approval rather than internal self-awareness.

This type of trauma is particularly difficult to recognize because it occurs within contexts that society views as privileged and successful. Alexandra struggles with guilt about her emotional difficulties because she "should" be grateful for her advantages. She minimizes her own suffering because it doesn't match societal definitions of trauma or neglect.

High-achieving families can inadvertently create environments where children develop quiet BPD through:

Enmeshment: Children become extensions of their parents' ambitions and identities rather than developing independent selves. Their achievements reflect on family status, creating pressure to maintain perfect external images.

Emotional substitution: Children learn to meet their parents' emotional needs rather than having their own needs met. They become the family therapist, cheerleader, or trophy, losing touch with their authentic emotional experiences.

Performance-based love: Affection and attention correlate directly with achievement and behavior. Children learn that love must be earned and can be withdrawn if they fail to meet expectations.

Perfectionist standards: Anything less than excellence is viewed as failure. Children develop all-or-nothing thinking patterns and learn to fear making mistakes or showing vulnerability.

The neurobiology of adaptation gone wrong

Research reveals that childhood experiences literally shape brain development, particularly in areas responsible for emotional regulation, stress response, and interpersonal attachment. Children who grow up with chronic emotional invalidation develop neurobiological patterns that persist into adulthood, creating the brain differences observed in BPD.

Rachel's developing brain adapted to her childhood environment by becoming hyper-vigilant to social threats and rejection. Her amygdala, responsible for threat detection, became highly sensitive to subtle signs of disapproval or abandonment. Simultaneously, her prefrontal cortex developed strong inhibitory control to suppress emotional expression that might result in rejection.

These adaptations made perfect sense in Rachel's childhood environment—they helped her maintain her parents' approval and avoid the distress of emotional invalidation. However, these same adaptations became problematic in adult relationships where emotional expression and vulnerability are necessary for genuine intimacy.

Dr. Allan Schore's research on attachment and brain development demonstrates that secure emotional relationships during childhood are necessary for healthy emotional regulation system development. Children who don't receive consistent emotional attunement and support develop dysregulated stress response systems that persist into adulthood.

The 40% heritability rate for BPD suggests that genetic factors contribute significantly to development, but environmental factors determine how genetic predispositions are expressed. A child born with genetic vulnerability to emotional dysregulation might develop healthy emotional regulation skills in a supportive environment or develop BPD symptoms in an invalidating environment.

Recognizing the perfect storm in your own history

Understanding the origins of quiet BPD can provide tremendous relief and insight, but it requires looking beyond obvious trauma to recognize subtler forms of emotional invalidation and neglect. Consider these patterns from your own childhood:

Emotional climate: Did your family openly discuss feelings, or were emotions treated as problems to solve quickly? Were you encouraged to express authentic emotions, or did you learn to suppress feelings that made others uncomfortable?

Achievement patterns: Did your parents' attention and approval correlate with your performance and behavior? Did you feel loved for who you were, or for what you accomplished?

Conflict resolution: How did your family handle disagreements and difficult emotions? Were conflicts addressed directly and respectfully, or avoided and swept under the rug?

Individual attention: Did your parents see and respond to you as a unique individual with your own needs and preferences, or did they expect you to fit into family expectations and roles?

Emotional support: When you felt scared, sad, or angry, did adults help you understand and process these emotions, or did they minimize, dismiss, or try to quickly fix your emotional experiences?

The path from understanding to healing

Rachel's advocacy work stems directly from her understanding of how quiet BPD develops. She recognizes that her parents weren't villains—they were doing their best with limited emotional skills and awareness. However, understanding the origins of her condition has helped her develop compassion for her own struggles while taking responsibility for her healing journey.

Recognition of quiet BPD's origins serves several important functions in recovery:

Reduces self-blame: Understanding that emotional dysregulation stems from understandable adaptations to childhood experiences helps reduce the shame and self-criticism that often accompany BPD.

Increases self-compassion: Recognizing that your emotional intensity and relationship patterns developed as protective responses to invalidating environments can help you treat yourself with greater kindness.

Informs treatment choices: Understanding your specific developmental history helps identify which therapeutic approaches might be most helpful and which relationship patterns need attention.

Guides family healing: If you have children, understanding how quiet BPD develops can help you provide the emotional support and validation that you didn't receive, potentially breaking intergenerational patterns.

Clarifies relationship dynamics: Understanding your childhood experiences helps you recognize how past patterns might be influencing current relationships and what changes might be helpful.

The goal isn't to blame parents or families for your struggles—most parents do their best with the skills and awareness they possess. Instead, the goal is to understand how your emotional patterns developed so you can make conscious choices about how to move forward in your healing journey.

Essential insights

Key understanding for quiet BPD origins and development:

- Childhood emotional neglect and invalidation, rather than obvious trauma, often contribute most significantly to quiet BPD development
- Highly sensitive children in emotionally invalidating environments are particularly vulnerable to developing internalized emotional dysregulation
- Intergenerational transmission of emotional suppression patterns means that loving parents can inadvertently contribute to quiet BPD development
- High-achieving families can create environments where children develop quiet BPD through performance-based love and perfectionist expectations
- Neurobiological adaptations to invalidating childhood environments persist into adulthood, creating the brain patterns observed in BPD

- Understanding developmental origins reduces self-blame, increases self-compassion, and informs effective treatment approaches
- Recognition of how quiet BPD develops can help break intergenerational patterns and improve current relationships

The next chapter will explore how quiet BPD often gets misdiagnosed, examining the complex process of accurate identification and the impact of missed or inappropriate diagnoses on treatment and recovery.

Chapter 4: The misdiagnosis maze

Jennifer's psychiatric records read like a medical mystery novel spanning fifteen years and seven different diagnoses. At nineteen, a college counselor diagnosed her with adjustment disorder after she sought help for what she described as "feeling overwhelmed." Three years later, an internist prescribed antidepressants for major depressive disorder after Jennifer reported persistent sadness and fatigue. By twenty-five, a psychiatrist had added generalized anxiety disorder to explain her constant worry and physical tension. A brief stint with an eating disorder specialist resulted in an EDNOS diagnosis. Later came social anxiety disorder, then complex PTSD after Jennifer disclosed childhood emotional neglect.

Each diagnosis captured part of Jennifer's experience but missed the underlying emotional dysregulation that drove all her symptoms. It wasn't until age thirty-four, when Jennifer finally found a clinician trained in quiet BPD presentations, that she received an accurate diagnosis that explained the complete picture of her mental health struggles. Jennifer's journey through the diagnostic maze illustrates one of the most challenging aspects of quiet BPD—its tendency to masquerade as other conditions, leading to years of ineffective treatment and continued suffering.

The labyrinth of overlapping symptoms

Quiet BPD presents a particular diagnostic challenge because its symptoms overlap significantly with numerous other mental health conditions. Unlike classic BPD, which includes dramatic behaviors that clearly indicate emotional dysregulation, quiet BPD symptoms often appear as standalone anxiety or mood disorders rather than expressions of underlying borderline dynamics.

Jennifer's depression wasn't simply major depressive disorder—it was the chronic emptiness and identity disturbance characteristic of BPD. Her anxiety wasn't generalized anxiety disorder—it was the intense fear of abandonment and rejection that drives BPD behaviors. Her eating disorder wasn't primarily about body image—it was a form of self-punishment and emotional regulation. Her social anxiety wasn't about general social situations—it was about the terror of being seen as defective or too much for others to handle.

The diagnostic confusion occurs because quiet BPD individuals often develop secondary conditions as attempts to manage their underlying emotional dysregulation. Jennifer's depression emerged from years of suppressing her authentic emotions and needs. Her anxiety developed from constantly monitoring others for signs of rejection. Her eating disorder became a way to channel self-punishment and achieve the control that felt impossible in emotional relationships.

Dr. Michael Chen, who specializes in complex diagnostic presentations, explains that quiet BPD often functions as the "root condition" that gives rise to other symptoms and diagnoses. Treating the secondary conditions without addressing the underlying emotional dysregulation often provides temporary relief but doesn't create lasting change because the root cause remains unaddressed.

Common misdiagnoses and their implications

Major Depressive Disorder represents the most frequent misdiagnosis for quiet BPD, particularly in individuals who present with chronic emptiness, persistent sadness, and feelings of worthlessness. However, BPD-related depression differs from major depression in several key ways:

- **Reactivity:** BPD depression often fluctuates rapidly based on interpersonal events, while major depression tends to be more stable and pervasive
- **Emptiness vs. sadness:** BPD individuals often describe feeling empty or hollow rather than sad, with brief moments of intense emotion punctuating long periods of numbness
- **Triggers:** BPD depression typically connects to relationship fears and identity confusion rather than the hopelessness and cognitive distortions of major depression

Sarah, a 28-year-old teacher, received antidepressant treatment for three years before anyone recognized that her "depression" was actually the chronic emptiness of quiet BPD. Her mood lifted temporarily with medication, but the underlying identity disturbance and relationship difficulties continued unchanged.

Generalized Anxiety Disorder also frequently overlaps with quiet BPD presentations, as both conditions involve persistent worry and physical anxiety symptoms. However, BPD anxiety focuses specifically on interpersonal threats and abandonment fears rather than general life concerns:

- **Content:** BPD anxiety centers on relationship security and self-worth, while GAD involves broader life concerns like health, finances, or general catastrophizing
- **Triggers:** BPD anxiety spikes with perceived rejection or criticism, while GAD maintains consistent levels regardless of interpersonal events
- **Physical symptoms:** BPD anxiety often includes dissociation and emotional numbness alongside traditional anxiety symptoms

Marcus discovered that his "generalized anxiety" was actually quiet BPD when he realized his worry focused almost exclusively on analyzing text messages, interpreting colleagues' facial expressions, and monitoring his girlfriend's mood changes for signs of potential rejection.

Complex PTSD shares many features with quiet BPD, including emotional dysregulation, identity disturbance, and relationship difficulties stemming from childhood experiences. The conditions often co-occur, making differential diagnosis particularly challenging:

- **Trauma focus:** C-PTSD symptoms typically connect directly to specific traumatic experiences, while BPD symptoms may persist even when trauma memories are processed

- **Identity patterns:** C-PTSD identity disturbance usually relates to trauma impacts, while BPD identity disturbance involves fundamental uncertainty about self-concept
- **Emotional regulation:** Both conditions involve dysregulation, but BPD emotional intensity often exceeds what would be expected from trauma history alone

Autism Spectrum Disorder occasionally gets confused with quiet BPD, particularly in women whose autism presentations don't match traditional male-centered diagnostic criteria. Both conditions can involve:

- Social difficulties and misreading interpersonal cues
- Intense emotional responses to environmental changes
- Need for routine and predictability
- Masking or camouflaging natural responses to appear socially acceptable

However, autism involves neurological differences in social communication and sensory processing, while quiet BPD involves emotional dysregulation and abandonment fears. Accurate differential diagnosis requires understanding whether social difficulties stem from neurological differences or emotional dysregulation patterns.

Gender bias in diagnostic patterns

Research consistently demonstrates that women receive BPD diagnoses at rates significantly higher than men, but this disparity reflects diagnostic bias rather than actual prevalence differences. Women's emotional expression tends to be more socially acceptable, making their BPD symptoms more visible to clinicians. Men's emotional dysregulation often gets channeled into behaviors that receive other diagnoses or no diagnosis at all.

David's quiet BPD manifested through workaholism, sexual compulsivity, and periodic alcohol binges—behaviors that didn't prompt mental health evaluation for years. When he finally sought treatment after a panic attack at work, clinicians focused on his anxiety symptoms and work stress rather than recognizing the underlying emotional dysregulation and identity disturbance that drove these surface behaviors.

Male socialization teaches emotional suppression from early childhood, making quiet BPD presentations even more likely in men than women. However, mental health professionals often miss these presentations because they don't match expected BPD symptoms and because men are less likely to seek help for emotional difficulties.

Women with quiet BPD face different challenges. Their emotional intensity might be dismissed as "normal" female emotionality, their people-pleasing seen as appropriate feminine behavior, and their perfectionism praised rather than recognized as symptoms of underlying distress. Female socialization that rewards emotional suppression and caretaking can mask quiet BPD symptoms as desirable feminine traits.

Age factors in recognition and diagnosis

Quiet BPD often emerges during adolescence but may not receive accurate diagnosis until midlife, particularly in high-functioning individuals who successfully mask their symptoms through achievement and external success. Different life stages present unique diagnostic challenges:

Adolescence and young adulthood: BPD symptoms during these developmental periods might be dismissed as "normal" teenage behavior or adjustment difficulties related to school transitions and relationship changes. However, adolescent quiet BPD often presents as perfectionism, social anxiety, and academic pressure rather than typical teenage rebellion.

Emma's parents attributed her high school emotional difficulties to "sensitivity" and "perfectionism," missing the intense fear of abandonment and identity confusion that drove her straight-A performance and people-pleasing behaviors. Her quiet BPD wasn't recognized until she experienced a severe depressive episode in

31

graduate school that finally prompted comprehensive mental health evaluation.

Middle age: Many individuals receive first-time quiet BPD diagnoses in their thirties, forties, or fifties when life stressors overwhelm their coping mechanisms or when they seek help for their children's emotional difficulties and recognize similar patterns in themselves.

Patricia, a 45-year-old executive, sought therapy after her teenage daughter was diagnosed with anxiety and depression. During family therapy sessions, Patricia recognized that her own childhood experiences and current emotional patterns matched many quiet BPD characteristics. Her high-functioning exterior had masked decades of internal emotional turmoil that she had attributed to "normal" stress and high achievement.

Later life: Older adults with undiagnosed quiet BPD might experience increased symptoms as retirement, health changes, or loss of loved ones disrupt the identity structures and coping mechanisms they've relied on for decades.

Clinical assessment challenges

Mental health professionals face several obstacles when assessing for quiet BPD, many stemming from training that emphasizes recognizing classic BPD presentations and the subtle nature of quiet BPD symptoms.

The "model patient" problem: Individuals with quiet BPD often present as ideal therapy clients—articulate, insightful, motivated, and compliant. They complete homework assignments thoroughly, arrive punctually, and provide detailed emotional descriptions. This presentation can mask the underlying emotional dysregulation because it doesn't match expectations of how BPD individuals behave in treatment.

Intellectualization vs. insight: Many quiet BPD individuals possess exceptional ability to analyze their emotional patterns and relationship dynamics. However, this intellectual understanding often serves as defense against actually feeling emotions rather than representing genuine insight or emotional processing.

High functioning masquerading as health: External success and achievement can mislead clinicians into underestimating internal distress levels. A client who maintains career success, stable relationships, and appropriate self-care might not seem to meet BPD severity criteria even when experiencing significant internal emotional chaos.

Therapeutic relationship dynamics: The therapeutic relationship itself becomes complicated with quiet BPD clients who are exquisitely sensitive to perceived rejection or criticism. They might carefully monitor their therapist's responses and adjust their presentations accordingly, making assessment more challenging.

Dr. Lisa Rodriguez, who trains clinicians in quiet BPD assessment, emphasizes the importance of looking beyond surface presentation to understand internal experiences: "We need to assess not just what clients are experiencing, but how much energy they're expending to maintain their functioning and what happens when their coping mechanisms are overwhelmed."

Family recognition challenges

Family members often struggle to recognize quiet BPD because the individual appears stable and successful from the outside. Parents might dismiss concerns as "sensitivity" or "perfectionism," while partners might not understand why someone so accomplished feels so insecure and emotionally needy.

Rebecca's husband couldn't understand why she obsessed over casual comments from friends, replayed conversations for hours, and seemed to need constant reassurance about their relationship despite his consistent demonstrations of love and commitment. Her quiet BPD symptoms were invisible to him because she managed to maintain her composure during most interactions, only revealing her emotional intensity in their private moments together.

Family education becomes particularly important for quiet BPD because loved ones need to understand that external success doesn't indicate emotional well-being and that the individual's need for reassurance and emotional support stems from neurobiological differences rather than character flaws or attention-seeking behaviors.

Signs that might alert family members to quiet BPD include:

- Disproportionate emotional responses to perceived criticism or rejection
- Excessive worry about relationships and others' opinions
- Perfectionist behaviors that cause distress rather than satisfaction
- Periods of emotional withdrawal following social interactions
- Difficulty making decisions without extensive reassurance
- Physical symptoms like headaches, stomach problems, or fatigue that worsen during interpersonal stress

The impact of misdiagnosis on treatment and recovery

Incorrect or incomplete diagnoses can significantly delay effective treatment and may actually worsen quiet BPD symptoms through inappropriate interventions. Jennifer's experience illustrates several common problems:

Medication trials that don't address core issues: Antidepressants and anti-anxiety medications might provide temporary symptom relief but don't address the underlying emotional dysregulation and identity disturbance that drive quiet BPD. Some individuals experience medication trials as evidence that they're "treatment-resistant" or that their problems are unfixable.

Therapy approaches that miss the mark: Traditional cognitive-behavioral therapy, while helpful for many conditions, might not address the deep-seated emotional regulation deficits and attachment patterns that characterize BPD. Clients might make intellectual progress while their emotional difficulties continue unchanged.

Self-blame and confusion: Multiple diagnoses and treatment failures often leave individuals feeling like they're "broken" or "too complicated" to help. They might blame themselves for not getting better despite trying multiple approaches.

Delayed access to effective treatments: Years of incorrect treatment delay access to specialized BPD interventions like dialectical behavior therapy (DBT) or mentalization-based therapy that could provide significant relief.

Financial and emotional costs: Multiple treatment attempts strain both financial resources and emotional resilience, sometimes leading individuals to give up on treatment entirely.

Creating pathways to accurate diagnosis

Accurate quiet BPD diagnosis requires clinicians trained in recognizing subtle presentations and clients who understand what symptoms to report. Several strategies can improve diagnostic accuracy:

Comprehensive assessment tools: Structured interviews and assessment instruments specifically designed for BPD can help identify symptoms that might be missed in traditional clinical interviews.

Longitudinal evaluation: Quiet BPD patterns become more apparent over time, particularly how emotional responses relate to interpersonal events and how identity disturbance manifests across different life domains.

Collateral information: Input from family members, partners, or close friends can provide valuable information about symptoms that individuals might not recognize or report themselves.

Trauma-informed assessment: Understanding childhood experiences and family dynamics helps contextualize current symptoms and identify developmental patterns consistent with BPD.

Differential diagnosis expertise: Clinicians need training in distinguishing BPD from other conditions that share similar symptoms, particularly complex trauma, autism spectrum disorders, and mood/anxiety disorders.

Essential insights

Key points for understanding quiet BPD misdiagnosis:

- Quiet BPD symptoms frequently overlap with depression, anxiety, PTSD, and other conditions, leading to years of incorrect treatment
- Gender bias affects diagnosis, with men's quiet BPD often going unrecognized and women's symptoms sometimes dismissed as normal emotional sensitivity
- Age factors influence recognition, with many individuals not receiving accurate diagnosis until midlife despite symptom onset in adolescence
- High-functioning presentations can mislead both clinicians and family members about symptom severity and treatment needs
- Misdiagnosis delays access to effective BPD treatments and may worsen symptoms through inappropriate interventions
- Accurate diagnosis requires specialized training, comprehensive assessment, and understanding of how quiet BPD differs from other mental health conditions
- Multiple failed treatments due to misdiagnosis can create additional trauma and self-blame that complicate recovery efforts

Chapter 5: Love in the shadows: Relationship patterns

M.K. first noticed the lotus tattoo on the soccer mom's wrist during a particularly heated parent meeting about fundraising goals. While other parents debated budget allocations with varying degrees of passion, this woman sat quietly in the back, contributing thoughtful suggestions when asked but never demanding attention. The delicate lotus design seemed incongruous with her conservative suburban appearance—SUV in the driveway, volunteer coordinator badge, perfectly coordinated activewear that suggested morning gym sessions before school drop-off.

Later, M.K. learned that Sarah had gotten the tattoo during what she called her "dark period"—six months when her marriage nearly ended, her anxiety reached unbearable levels, and she finally sought therapy after years of appearing to manage everything perfectly. The lotus represented her decision to stop pretending she didn't struggle, to acknowledge that beauty could emerge from muddy waters, and to begin the difficult work of creating authentic relationships instead of performing for others' approval.

Sarah's story illustrates the complex relationship dynamics that characterize quiet BPD—the exhausting dance of craving connection while simultaneously building walls to protect against rejection, the tendency to lose oneself in relationships while fearing intimacy, and the challenge of maintaining relationships when your emotional reality remains largely invisible to others.

The dance of approach and avoidance

Relationships represent both the greatest source of healing and the most significant trigger for individuals with quiet BPD. The same emotional intensity that makes deep connections possible also creates overwhelming fears about vulnerability, rejection, and abandonment. This creates what clinicians call the "approach-avoidance" pattern—

desperately wanting closeness while simultaneously engaging in behaviors that create distance.

Sarah's marriage exemplified this dynamic. She craved emotional intimacy with her husband David but found actual vulnerability terrifying. She would hint at her emotional needs through subtle comments or behaviors, hoping he would notice and respond without her having to ask directly. When he missed these indirect communications—as most partners do—she would interpret his response as evidence that he didn't really care about her emotional world.

The approach behaviors in quiet BPD relationships often include:

Subtle testing: Making indirect comments or creating small situations to gauge a partner's commitment or emotional availability. Sarah might mention feeling tired or stressed and monitor David's response for evidence of care and attention.

Hypervigilant care: Anticipating and meeting a partner's needs in hopes of receiving similar attention. Sarah tracked David's preferences, moods, and schedules with remarkable accuracy, hoping he would reciprocate this level of attention to her emotional state.

Emotional breadcrumbs: Dropping hints about deeper struggles or needs without explicitly stating them. Sarah might mention having a "rough day" while hoping David would probe deeper and discover her underlying emotional distress.

Performance of stability: Working overtime to appear emotionally stable and independent to avoid burdening the relationship while secretly longing for someone to see through the facade and offer support.

The avoidance behaviors often emerge when vulnerability feels too dangerous:

Emotional withdrawal: Retreating into self-sufficiency when feeling too emotionally exposed. After sharing a vulnerable moment with David, Sarah might become distant and independent for several days, protecting herself from potential rejection.

Preemptive rejection: Creating reasons to end relationships or create distance before the other person can reject them first. Sarah would sometimes pick fights or create drama when she felt too dependent on David's love and support.

Minimizing needs: Downplaying emotional distress or relationship concerns to avoid appearing "too needy" or demanding. Sarah would often say she was "fine" even when experiencing significant internal turmoil.

Perfectionist maintenance: Focusing on external relationship management—keeping the house perfect, planning elaborate dates, managing social calendars—rather than addressing emotional intimacy.

Silent storms versus explosive eruptions

One of the most distinctive features of quiet BPD in relationships is how conflict gets handled. Unlike classic BPD presentations that might involve dramatic arguments, threats, or explosive emotional displays, quiet BPD individuals often internalize relationship conflicts, creating silent storms that partners may not even recognize.

David learned to dread the quiet periods more than arguments. When Sarah felt hurt or angry, she would become perfectly polite, efficient, and distant. She would continue managing household tasks, attending social events, and maintaining external appearances while internally experiencing emotional hurricanes. Her anger turned inward, becoming self-criticism and depression rather than outward expressions that David could recognize and respond to.

This pattern creates unique relationship challenges:

Invisible conflict: Partners often don't realize that conflicts are occurring because the quiet BPD individual doesn't express anger or hurt directly. David would sometimes discover days later that Sarah had been upset about something he had said or done, leaving him feeling confused and frustrated that she hadn't simply told him about the problem when it occurred.

Accumulated resentment: Without direct communication about problems, small issues accumulate into larger relationship wounds. Sarah would silently catalog perceived slights or disappointments until they became major relationship themes in her mind, even though David remained unaware of most individual incidents.

Emotional detective work: Partners may find themselves constantly trying to decode mood changes, subtle behavioral shifts, and indirect communications to understand their loved one's emotional state. David became hypervigilant to Sarah's subtle cues, trying to anticipate problems before they resulted in emotional withdrawal.

Resolution difficulties: Since conflicts aren't acknowledged directly, they rarely get resolved completely. Issues tend to resurface repeatedly because the underlying emotional dynamics haven't been addressed through open communication.

When quiet BPD individuals do express anger or frustration directly, it often comes after long periods of suppression and may feel disproportionate to the immediate trigger. Sarah's rare outbursts would confuse David because they seemed to involve issues he thought had been resolved or that seemed minor in the moment, not understanding that she was expressing accumulated emotions from multiple incidents.

The "too much" belief system

Perhaps the most destructive relationship pattern in quiet BPD involves the core belief that one's authentic emotional self is "too much" for others to handle. This belief system, usually developed during childhood experiences of emotional invalidation, creates self-fulfilling prophecies that sabotage relationships even when partners are willing and able to provide emotional support.

Sarah's "too much" beliefs manifested in several ways:

Emotional rationing: She carefully monitored how much emotional support she requested from David, keeping internal tallies of how often she had shared difficulties or asked for comfort. She would force herself to appear cheerful and independent even when struggling, believing that showing too much need would overwhelm or burden him.

Preemptive apologizing: She would apologize for her emotions before expressing them, framing her needs as inconveniences or burdens. "I'm sorry to bother you with this, but..." became a standard preface to any vulnerable sharing.

Emotional perfectionism: She expected herself to handle most emotional difficulties independently and felt guilty when she needed support. Her internalized message was that "good" partners don't require much emotional caretaking and that needing comfort or reassurance indicated personal weakness.

Hyperanalysis of responses: She would scrutinize David's responses to her emotional needs for any signs of annoyance, boredom, or withdrawal. A momentary distraction or slightly different tone would be interpreted as evidence that she had indeed been "too much."

This belief system creates relationship dynamics where partners can't win—they don't receive honest communication about their loved one's emotional needs, but they also get criticized (internally if not openly) for not providing adequate support. David found himself in the impossible position of trying to guess Sarah's needs while being given subtle messages that having needs in the first place was problematic.

The "too much" belief also prevents individuals from discovering that many partners are actually capable of handling emotional intensity and would welcome more authentic communication. Sarah never gave

41

David the opportunity to demonstrate that he could handle her emotional complexity because she edited herself so heavily before sharing anything with him.

Intimacy fears and emotional shapeshifting

Genuine intimacy requires showing your authentic self to another person and believing they will accept you as you are. For individuals with quiet BPD, this level of vulnerability feels extremely dangerous because their sense of self often depends on others' approval and acceptance. This creates what Dr. Amanda Johnson calls "intimacy paradox"—craving closeness while fearing the authenticity that real closeness requires.

Sarah dealt with intimacy fears through emotional shapeshifting—constantly adjusting her personality, opinions, and emotional expressions based on what she believed David wanted to see. She became skilled at reading his moods and preferences, then presenting versions of herself that would maintain his approval and affection.

This pattern showed up in numerous ways:

Opinion morphing: Sarah would subtly align her views with David's on everything from political issues to restaurant preferences, often without realizing she was doing it. She would genuinely believe she shared his preferences because she had suppressed her own opinions so completely.

Emotional mirroring: She would match David's emotional tone and energy level, becoming cheerful when he was upbeat and subdued when he seemed stressed. Her own emotional state became secondary to maintaining emotional harmony in the relationship.

Interest adoption: Sarah would enthusiastically embrace David's hobbies and interests while neglecting her own. She became knowledgeable about sports, invested in his work projects, and supportive of his social activities while her own interests faded into the background.

Personality adaptation: Around David's friends, she would emphasize different aspects of her personality than she showed around her own friends or family, creating multiple versions of herself for different social contexts.

This shapeshifting served short-term relationship maintenance but prevented genuine intimacy from developing. David fell in love with Sarah's presentation of herself rather than her authentic self, while Sarah never discovered what it felt like to be loved for who she really was. The relationship felt unstable to both of them because it was based on performance rather than genuine connection.

Splitting in silence

The psychological defense mechanism of splitting—seeing people as either all good or all bad—operates differently in quiet BPD than in classic presentations. Instead of dramatically idealizing and devaluing partners externally, quiet BPD individuals often experience these shifts internally while maintaining stable external behavior toward the relationship.

Sarah's internal experience of David would fluctuate dramatically based on relatively minor interactions. When he remembered to ask about her day or showed affection spontaneously, she would feel flooded with gratitude and love, internally idealizing him as the perfect, understanding partner. When he seemed distracted during conversations or forgot something she had mentioned, she would swing to the opposite extreme, seeing him as selfish and uncaring.

These internal splitting episodes caused significant relationship distress:

Emotional whiplash: Sarah would experience intense emotional reactions to David's behavior that felt disproportionate even to her. She might feel devastated by a brief comment that he made thoughtlessly, then feel guilty for overreacting while still experiencing the intense emotional pain.

Relationship paranoia: During "all bad" episodes, Sarah would interpret David's neutral behaviors as evidence of problems in their relationship. His choice to read instead of talking would become proof that he was withdrawing from her, rather than simply being tired after work.

Secret keeping: Unlike classic BPD presentations where splitting might result in dramatic confrontations or relationship chaos, Sarah would hide these internal experiences from David. She would maintain surface-level relationship functioning while privately experiencing intense emotional turmoil about their connection.

Recovery confusion: When splitting episodes resolved and Sarah returned to seeing David more realistically, she would feel confused about her previous intense reactions and might dismiss her concerns as "overreacting" rather than recognizing them as symptoms needing attention.

David remained largely unaware of Sarah's internal splitting episodes, but he sensed underlying tension and emotional distance that he couldn't identify or address. Sarah's ability to hide her splitting actually prevented David from understanding her struggles and offering appropriate support.

Building authentic connection

Recovery from quiet BPD relationship patterns requires learning to tolerate the vulnerability that authentic relationships require while developing skills to communicate emotional needs directly and effectively. Sarah's journey toward healthier relationships involved several key realizations and skill developments:

Recognizing emotional editing: Sarah had to become aware of how much she censored herself before sharing thoughts and feelings with David. She began noticing when she edited comments to make them more palatable or when she suppressed reactions to avoid potential conflict.

Practicing direct communication: Instead of hoping David would notice her indirect hints, Sarah learned to express her needs and feelings clearly. This felt terrifying initially because it meant risking direct rejection, but it also allowed David to respond appropriately to her actual needs rather than trying to guess what she wanted.

Tolerating relationship imperfection: Sarah had to accept that David couldn't meet all her emotional needs perfectly and that this didn't mean he didn't care about her. She learned to distinguish between David's limitations and evidence of rejection or abandonment.

Developing emotional self-soothing: Rather than depending entirely on David's responses to regulate her emotions, Sarah learned techniques to manage emotional storms independently. This reduced the pressure on their relationship while building her confidence in her ability to handle difficult emotions.

Creating space for authenticity: Sarah began sharing her interests, opinions, and preferences even when they differed from David's. She discovered that their relationship actually became stronger when she brought her authentic self to their interactions.

Key understanding of quiet BPD relationship patterns:

- Quiet BPD creates approach-avoidance dynamics where individuals crave intimacy while fearing the vulnerability that authentic connection requires
- Conflict often gets internalized rather than expressed, creating silent emotional storms that partners may not recognize or understand
- Core beliefs about being "too much" for others prevent authentic communication and create self-fulfilling prophecies about relationship rejection
- Intimacy fears lead to emotional shapeshifting and people-pleasing that prevents genuine connection from developing
- Splitting occurs internally rather than through dramatic external behaviors, causing intense private emotional experiences that partners may not witness

45

- Recovery involves learning direct communication, tolerating vulnerability, and bringing authentic self-expression to relationships
- Partners benefit from education about quiet BPD patterns and learning to recognize subtle signs of emotional distress

The next chapter will examine how quiet BPD affects professional life and achievement, exploring the complex relationship between perfectionism, success, and internal emotional struggles in work environments.

Chapter 6: Success and suffering: Work and achievement

Gary's pattern became clear only in retrospect. Three years at the consulting firm, followed by a sudden resignation citing "better opportunities." Two and a half years at the tech startup, until conflicts with management made the environment "untenable." Three years at the marketing agency before a reorganization made him decide the culture "no longer aligned" with his values. Each transition seemed logical and career-advancing from the outside. Each departure followed the same internal pattern—initial enthusiasm and exceptional performance, growing perfectionist demands on himself, increasing anxiety about perceived criticism, and eventual burnout that made staying impossible.

Now thirty-five and contemplating yet another job change, Gary finally recognized the pattern that had shaped his entire professional life. His quiet BPD didn't just affect his personal relationships—it created a complex dance with achievement and professional identity that left him successful on paper but perpetually exhausted and unsatisfied in reality.

Perfectionism as emotional armor

For many individuals with quiet BPD, professional achievement serves a dual purpose: it provides external validation that temporarily soothes internal feelings of inadequacy, and it creates a competent facade that masks emotional vulnerability from colleagues and supervisors. Gary's exceptional work performance wasn't simply about professional ambition—it was emotional armor designed to protect against criticism and rejection.

Gary's perfectionism manifested in ways that initially impressed employers but ultimately created unsustainable work patterns:

Excessive preparation: Gary would spend hours researching topics for meetings, creating detailed backup plans for presentations, and anticipating every possible question or criticism. While colleagues might prepare for thirty minutes, Gary would invest entire evenings ensuring his contribution was flawless.

Invisible overtime: Gary regularly arrived early and stayed late, not because he had too much work but because he couldn't bear the possibility of submitting anything less than perfect. He would revise reports multiple times, restructure presentations repeatedly, and double-check work that colleagues would consider finished after the first draft.

Hypervigilant monitoring: Gary constantly scanned his work environment for signs of approval or disapproval. A supervisor's neutral expression during his presentation would trigger hours of internal analysis about what he might have done wrong. Positive feedback never felt sufficient—it was either insincere politeness or would quickly be overshadowed by worry about maintaining the same standard.

Preventive overwork: Gary would take on additional projects and responsibilities, not from enthusiasm but from fear that saying no would be interpreted as laziness or lack of commitment. His workload became overwhelming, but reducing it felt like admitting incompetence.

This perfectionist armor served its protective function—Gary rarely received direct criticism because his work quality was genuinely exceptional. However, the emotional cost was enormous. He lived in constant fear of making mistakes, experienced work as perpetually stressful rather than satisfying, and could never enjoy his achievements because he was already worried about the next potential failure.

Imposter syndrome on steroids

Most professionals experience occasional self-doubt about their abilities or worry about being exposed as less competent than others believe. For individuals with quiet BPD, these feelings intensify into persistent, overwhelming imposter syndrome that no amount of external success can alleviate.

Gary's imposter syndrome extended far beyond normal professional insecurities. Despite consistent positive performance reviews, promotions, and recognition from supervisors and colleagues, he remained convinced that he was fundamentally incompetent and that others would eventually discover his "fraud." His internal experience bore no relationship to external evidence of his abilities.

The intensity of quiet BPD imposter syndrome stems from several factors:

Identity instability: Without a stable sense of self, professional identity becomes entirely dependent on others' perceptions and reactions. Gary never felt like he "was" a skilled professional—he felt like he was successfully pretending to be one, with constant risk of exposure.

All-or-nothing thinking: Small mistakes or areas of uncertainty became evidence of complete incompetence. When Gary didn't know the answer to a question during a meeting, he interpreted this as proof that he was unqualified for his position, rather than recognizing that no one knows everything about their field.

Achievement discounting: Gary would attribute successes to luck, timing, or other external factors while viewing mistakes as evidence of his true incompetence. Positive feedback felt unearned or based on incomplete information about his abilities.

Constant comparison: Gary measured himself against idealized versions of colleagues, assuming others felt confident and competent in ways that he never experienced. He didn't recognize that many colleagues shared similar insecurities because they, like him, hid their doubts behind professional facades.

Perfectionist standards: Gary's internal standards for competence were impossibly high. He believed he should know everything, never

49

make mistakes, and handle all situations with ease. Normal learning curves and professional challenges felt like personal failures rather than typical aspects of career development.

This persistent imposter syndrome created work environments where Gary never felt safe or secure, regardless of his actual performance quality. Success provided only temporary relief from his fears of inadequacy, and each new challenge triggered fresh waves of anxiety about potential exposure.

When burnout becomes a repetitive cycle

Gary's job transitions weren't random career changes—they were burnout cycles driven by the unsustainable emotional demands of maintaining perfectionist performance while managing internal emotional storms. The pattern repeated with each new position because Gary never addressed the underlying emotional dynamics that created the burnout in the first place.

The cycle typically unfolded in predictable stages:

Honeymoon phase: Each new job began with enthusiasm and hope. Gary felt energized by the fresh start, new challenges, and opportunity to prove himself in a different environment. His perfectionist tendencies would initially be sustainable and even advantageous as he learned new systems and impressed supervisors with his thoroughness.

Escalation phase: As Gary became more comfortable in the role, expectations increased—both from supervisors and from himself. Projects became more complex, deadlines more demanding, and stakes higher. Gary would respond by intensifying his perfectionist behaviors, working longer hours and becoming more anxious about potential mistakes.

Crisis phase: Eventually, the combination of perfectionist demands and emotional dysregulation would become overwhelming. Gary would experience physical symptoms—headaches, insomnia, digestive problems—alongside increased emotional volatility. Small workplace conflicts would feel catastrophic, and criticism would trigger days of rumination and self-attack.

Escape phase: Rather than addressing the underlying patterns, Gary would begin planning his exit. He would rationalize leaving as a career advancement opportunity or cultural mismatch, not recognizing that his internal emotional dynamics were creating the workplace difficulties he was trying to escape.

Recovery phase: The period between jobs provided temporary relief from workplace stressors, allowing Gary to feel optimistic about his next position. This recovery phase reinforced his belief that the problems had been with the specific workplace rather than his own emotional patterns.

This cycle created several long-term career problems:

Skill development limitations: Constant job changes prevented Gary from developing deep expertise or building long-term professional relationships that could support career advancement.

Pattern recognition avoidance: Each move allowed Gary to avoid examining his contribution to workplace difficulties, maintaining the illusion that external factors were responsible for his professional struggles.

Increasing anxiety: With each repetition of the cycle, Gary became more anxious about his ability to maintain any job long-term, creating additional pressure that accelerated the burnout timeline.

Identity confusion: Without sustained success in any single role, Gary struggled to develop a coherent professional identity or confidence in his career direction.

Executive function struggles behind the facade

While Gary appeared highly organized and competent to colleagues, he privately struggled with executive functioning challenges that required enormous mental energy to manage. The emotional dysregulation of quiet BPD often impairs cognitive functions like attention, working memory, and decision-making, even when these difficulties aren't visible to others.

Gary's executive function struggles included:

Decision paralysis: Simple work decisions became overwhelming when Gary considered all possible outcomes and their potential for criticism. Choosing which approach to take on a project might consume hours of internal debate, with Gary researching multiple options extensively before making choices that colleagues would make intuitively.

Attention fragmentation: While Gary could hyperfocus on projects that captured his interest, routine tasks often suffered from attention difficulties. His mind would wander to relationship concerns, self-critical thoughts, or anxiety about future challenges, making it hard to concentrate on mundane but necessary work.

Working memory interference: Emotional preoccupations would interfere with Gary's ability to hold multiple pieces of information in mind simultaneously. During complex meetings or when juggling multiple projects, his cognitive resources would be divided between work tasks and emotional regulation, reducing his effective mental capacity.

Planning and prioritization challenges: Gary would create elaborate systems for organizing his work but struggle to implement them consistently when emotional stress increased. He might spend more time perfecting his organizational system than actually completing the work it was designed to manage.

Cognitive flexibility problems: When initial approaches to problems didn't work, Gary would become stuck rather than easily shifting to alternative strategies. His perfectionist mindset made it difficult to abandon approaches he had invested time in, even when they weren't producing results.

These executive function challenges remained largely invisible because Gary compensated through overwork and excessive preparation. He would arrive early to gather his thoughts, create detailed notes to support his memory, and build extra time into all projects to accommodate his inefficiencies. Colleagues saw the results—high-quality work delivered on time—without recognizing the tremendous effort required to produce them.

The performance trap

Gary's professional success created what therapists call the "performance trap"—external achievements that reinforce internal beliefs about conditional worth while preventing the authentic self-expression that could lead to genuine satisfaction and sustainable success.

The trap operated through several mechanisms:

Validation addiction: Each professional success provided temporary relief from feelings of inadequacy, creating a cycle where Gary needed increasingly impressive achievements to feel worthy. Promotions, awards, and recognition became drugs that temporarily numbed his internal pain without addressing underlying emotional wounds.

Authentic self suppression: Gary's professional persona bore little resemblance to his authentic personality and interests. He had learned to emphasize aspects of himself that seemed valuable to employers while hiding qualities that felt too risky or vulnerable to reveal. This created a professional life that felt like constant acting.

Success anxiety: Paradoxically, Gary's achievements increased rather than decreased his anxiety. Each success raised expectations and stakes, making future failures feel more catastrophic. Success became a burden rather than a reward.

Identity fusion: Gary's sense of self became entirely dependent on professional achievement. When work went well, he felt valuable and competent. When work challenges arose, his entire self-worth collapsed. This created enormous pressure on his career to provide not just income but complete identity validation.

Relationship avoidance: Gary's focus on achievement allowed him to avoid the interpersonal vulnerability that his quiet BPD made terrifying. Work relationships remained professional and safe, protecting him from the emotional risks of deeper connections while reinforcing his isolation.

The performance trap is particularly insidious because it's socially reinforced. Family, friends, and society applaud professional achievement, making it difficult for individuals to recognize when success is serving psychological avoidance rather than genuine fulfillment.

Workplace relationship dynamics

Gary's quiet BPD significantly affected his workplace relationships, though colleagues rarely recognized the underlying emotional dynamics. His interpersonal patterns at work mirrored those in his personal life—intense fear of rejection and criticism masked by competent, helpful behavior that kept others at arm's length.

Colleague relationships: Gary maintained friendly but superficial relationships with coworkers. He was known as reliable, helpful, and easy to work with, but no one knew him personally. He would remember colleagues' birthdays, offer assistance with projects, and participate in social events, but never shared personal struggles or authentic emotions.

Authority relationships: Interactions with supervisors triggered Gary's most intense BPD symptoms. He would obsessively analyze feedback for signs of disapproval, interpret neutral comments as criticism, and adjust his behavior based on subtle cues about supervisors' preferences. His exceptional attention to authority figures' needs made him valuable to managers but exhausted him emotionally.

Team dynamics: Gary often became the unofficial emotional caretaker for work teams, sensing tension and working to smooth over conflicts before they became disruptive. This role felt familiar from his childhood experiences managing family emotions, but it prevented him from focusing on his own work responsibilities and career development.

Conflict avoidance: Gary would go to great lengths to avoid workplace conflicts, often taking on additional work or accepting unreasonable demands rather than setting appropriate boundaries. When conflicts were unavoidable, he would internalize stress rather than addressing issues directly, leading to physical and emotional symptoms.

Recognition patterns: Gary's need for validation made him highly sensitive to recognition and praise, but he couldn't accept positive feedback as genuine. He would discount compliments, assume they were motivated by politeness rather than sincerity, and continue working to "earn" the approval he had already received.

Creating sustainable professional relationships

Gary's recognition of his quiet BPD patterns opened the door to developing a more sustainable and authentic relationship with work and professional achievement. This process required distinguishing between genuine career interests and BPD-driven perfectionism while learning to find satisfaction in work without depending on it for complete identity validation.

Authentic interest exploration: Gary began examining which aspects of his work genuinely engaged him versus which activities he pursued primarily for external validation. He discovered interests in mentoring junior colleagues and strategic planning that he had previously overlooked in favor of more prestigious but less personally meaningful projects.

Boundary development: Gary learned to set appropriate limits on his work hours and project commitments. This felt terrifying initially because he feared disappointing supervisors, but he discovered that working more sustainably actually improved his performance quality and creativity.

Feedback reframing: With therapeutic support, Gary developed skills to interpret workplace feedback more realistically. He learned to distinguish between constructive criticism meant to help him improve and evidence of personal inadequacy or job insecurity.

Relationship authenticity: Gary began sharing appropriate personal information with trusted colleagues, moving beyond surface-level professional relationships toward genuine workplace friendships. This increased his job satisfaction while providing social support during stressful periods.

Success redefinition: Gary worked to define professional success in terms of personal growth, skill development, and contribution to meaningful projects rather than purely external measures like promotions or salary increases. This reduced the pressure on his career to provide complete identity validation.

Emotional regulation at work: Gary developed strategies for managing emotional triggers in workplace settings—taking brief breaks when feeling overwhelmed, using breathing techniques during stressful meetings, and creating end-of-day rituals to transition from work to personal life.

Key understanding of quiet BPD in professional settings:

- Perfectionism in quiet BPD serves as emotional armor against criticism and rejection but creates unsustainable work patterns and chronic stress
- Imposter syndrome intensifies beyond normal professional insecurities, creating persistent feelings of fraudulence regardless of actual achievement levels
- Burnout cycles repeat across different jobs because underlying emotional patterns remain unaddressed, leading to frequent career transitions

- Executive function struggles remain hidden behind competent facades but require enormous mental energy to manage effectively
- Professional success can create performance traps that reinforce conditional self-worth while preventing authentic self-expression
- Workplace relationships mirror personal relationship patterns, involving fear-based people-pleasing and emotional caretaking of colleagues
- Sustainable professional life requires distinguishing between genuine interests and BPD-driven achievement while developing authentic workplace relationships

The next chapter will explore the daily reality of living with quiet BPD, examining the internal struggles that others rarely see and the practical challenges of managing emotional storms while maintaining external composure.

Chapter 7: The daily battle no one sees

The cereal aisle shouldn't be this complicated. Standing in front of thirty different breakfast options, Maria feels her chest tighten with the familiar weight of decision paralysis. Cheerios or granola? The healthy choice would be steel-cut oats, but that requires planning ahead. Instant oatmeal seems lazy. The organic options cost more—is she worth the extra expense? Each choice carries invisible emotional weight, connecting to deeper questions about self-worth, responsibility, and what kind of person she's supposed to be.

Twenty minutes later, Maria leaves the store with nothing, overwhelmed by the cascading thoughts and emotional reactions that a simple breakfast choice triggered. To anyone observing, she might appear indecisive or particular about food. They couldn't see the internal storm of self-judgment, the exhaustion from analyzing every option for its implications about her character, or the shame about being unable to handle what others do effortlessly.

This scene repeats daily in countless variations for people with quiet BPD—moments when routine decisions become emotional minefields, when maintaining external composure requires tremendous internal effort, and when the gap between how others perceive you and how you experience yourself feels impossibly wide.

Decision paralysis in a world of choices

For individuals with quiet BPD, decision-making activates the same neurobiological systems involved in threat detection and emotional dysregulation. What appears as simple choice-making to others becomes complex emotional processing about identity, worth, and potential consequences that feel far more significant than the actual decision warrants.

Maria's cereal dilemma illustrates several factors that make routine decisions overwhelming for people with quiet BPD:

Identity uncertainty: Without a stable sense of self, every choice becomes a question about who you're supposed to be. Does buying expensive organic food mean you're pretentious? Does choosing generic brands mean you don't value yourself? The cereal choice becomes a referendum on personal identity rather than simply a preference for taste or nutrition.

Perfectionist analysis: Each option gets evaluated for its potential to be the "wrong" choice. Maria considers nutritional content, cost-effectiveness, environmental impact, and social implications of her selection. The decision-making process becomes exhaustive because every factor feels equally important and failure to consider all angles feels irresponsible.

Rejection sensitivity: Choices carry the weight of potential judgment from others. Maria worries that her selection might be criticized by checkout clerks, family members who see her pantry, or herself during future moments of self-reflection. The fear of making choices that others might disapprove of makes even mundane decisions feel risky.

Emotional forecasting errors: Maria attempts to predict how each choice will make her feel in the future, but her emotional prediction skills are impaired by the intensity and instability of her emotional responses. She can't reliably know if she'll feel satisfied or regretful about any option, making the decision process feel like gambling with her emotional well-being.

Executive function overload: The cognitive resources required to manage emotional regulation while making decisions leave fewer mental resources available for the decision-making process itself. Maria's brain is simultaneously trying to choose breakfast and manage anxiety about the choice, creating cognitive interference that makes thinking clearly more difficult.

This decision paralysis extends far beyond grocery stores. People with quiet BPD often struggle with:

- Choosing restaurants when dining with friends

- Selecting clothes for social events
- Deciding how to respond to text messages
- Picking movies or entertainment options
- Making weekend plans or vacation arrangements
- Choosing gifts for others
- Deciding when to leave social gatherings

Each choice activates the same internal systems, creating daily life that feels emotionally exhausting rather than routine.

The chameleon effect: Identity shapeshifting

Perhaps no aspect of daily life with quiet BPD is more exhausting than the constant monitoring and adjustment of self-presentation based on social context and others' apparent expectations. This "chameleon effect" represents an attempt to maintain connection and approval by becoming whatever others seem to want, but it comes at the cost of authentic self-knowledge and genuine relationships.

David's day illustrates this pattern in action. At his morning coffee shop, he's the friendly regular who knows the baristas' names and makes pleasant small talk about weekend plans. During his commute, he transforms into the efficient professional, checking emails and mentally preparing for meetings. At work, he becomes the collaborative team member who agrees with supervisors' ideas and offers helpful suggestions. During lunch with colleagues, he's the interested listener who asks thoughtful questions about others' projects. At happy hour, he's the easygoing friend who goes along with group decisions about venues and activities.

Each transformation feels natural in the moment, but David experiences emotional exhaustion from constantly monitoring and adjusting his presentation. By evening, he struggles to remember what he actually thinks about the topics discussed throughout the day or what his authentic preferences might be for how to spend his time.

The chameleon effect involves several automatic processes:

Emotional mirroring: Unconsciously matching others' emotional tone and energy levels. David becomes enthusiastic when others seem excited, serious when they appear concerned, and relaxed when they seem casual. This mirroring happens so automatically that he often doesn't realize he's doing it.

Opinion alignment: Adjusting viewpoints and preferences to match what others seem to value. David finds himself agreeing with political opinions, entertainment preferences, and lifestyle choices that don't necessarily reflect his own values or interests.

Personality emphasis: Highlighting different aspects of his personality depending on social context. David emphasizes his analytical skills with some colleagues, his creative interests with others, and his social abilities with friends, presenting different facets of himself as complete pictures.

Interest adoption: Developing enthusiasm for activities, topics, or hobbies that others find interesting. David has accumulated knowledge about sports, music, movies, and cultural events primarily to maintain conversations rather than from genuine personal interest.

Style adaptation: Changing communication patterns, humor styles, and social behaviors to match different groups. David speaks more formally with some colleagues, uses different humor with different friend groups, and adjusts his social energy level based on others' apparent preferences.

This constant adaptation serves the protective function of maintaining social acceptance and avoiding rejection, but it prevents David from developing a coherent sense of self or experiencing relationships based on authentic connection.

Managing emotional hurricanes in silence

The most invisible aspect of quiet BPD involves the internal emotional storms that occur regularly while maintaining external composure. These emotional experiences can be intense enough to feel

61

overwhelming and disruptive, yet others remain unaware that anything significant is happening internally.

Sarah's afternoon provides an example of this dynamic. During a team meeting, her supervisor makes a casual comment about deadlines that Sarah interprets as criticism of her time management. While continuing to participate normally in the meeting—asking appropriate questions, taking notes, contributing to discussions—Sarah experiences internal emotional chaos that includes racing thoughts about her competence, physical anxiety symptoms, shame about her perceived inadequacy, and fears about job security.

The emotional storm continues for hours after the meeting, with Sarah analyzing every aspect of the interaction while managing her regular work responsibilities. She completes emails, attends other meetings, and maintains professional relationships while simultaneously experiencing what feels like emotional crisis.

This pattern of internal emotional intensity alongside external functionality creates several unique challenges:

Delayed processing: Because emotional reactions must be suppressed during social interactions, processing often gets delayed until private moments. Sarah might not fully experience the impact of workplace events until evening, when she finally has space to feel without maintaining professional composure.

Cumulative exhaustion: Managing emotional storms while maintaining functionality requires enormous energy. Sarah feels drained at the end of workdays not just from professional responsibilities but from the effort required to regulate her emotional responses while continuing to perform effectively.

Validation confusion: When others don't recognize the significance of emotional triggers, it becomes difficult to know if reactions are proportionate or excessive. Sarah questions whether her supervisor's comment warranved her intense response, but has no external feedback to help calibrate her emotional reactions.

Support system gaps: Because the emotional struggles remain invisible, Sarah doesn't receive comfort or support during difficult moments. Others can't offer help when they don't know help is needed, leaving her to manage intense emotions without social support.

Recovery uncertainty: Without external validation of emotional experiences, it becomes difficult to know when emotions have been processed adequately. Sarah might continue ruminating about workplace interactions because she hasn't received confirmation that her concerns are valid or that the situation has been resolved.

Social exhaustion and the recovery cocoon

Social interactions, even positive ones, require tremendous energy for individuals with quiet BPD because each interaction involves emotional regulation, self-monitoring, and performance of appropriate social behaviors while managing internal emotional responses to subtle social cues.

After social events, many people with quiet BPD require extended periods of solitude to recover from the emotional and cognitive demands of social interaction. This recovery period might be misunderstood by others as antisocial behavior or lack of interest in relationships, when it's actually necessary emotional self-care.

Jennifer's weekend illustrates this pattern. After attending a friend's birthday party Saturday evening—where she appeared social, engaged, and cheerful—she spends most of Sunday alone in her apartment, declining invitations and avoiding phone calls. During the party, she monitored her facial expressions, analyzed conversations for social cues, managed anxiety about her appearance and social performance, and regulated her emotional responses to various interactions.

Sunday becomes her recovery day, where she:

Processes social interactions: Replaying conversations to analyze what went well and what might have been problematic. Jennifer reviews her social performance, looking for evidence that she made mistakes or that others viewed her negatively.

Regulates delayed emotions: Feelings that were suppressed during social interactions emerge when she's finally alone. Jennifer might feel sad about a comment someone made, anxious about a perceived social misstep, or overwhelmed by the emotional intensity of group dynamics.

Restores energy resources: The cognitive and emotional demands of social masking leave Jennifer feeling depleted. Solitude provides opportunity to rest without monitoring others' needs or maintaining appropriate social presentation.

Reconnects with authentic self: After hours of adapting to social expectations, Jennifer needs time to remember her own thoughts, feelings, and preferences. The recovery period allows her to distinguish between her authentic responses and her social performance.

Prepares for future interactions: Jennifer uses alone time to mentally prepare for upcoming social obligations, planning conversation topics, anticipating potential challenges, and building emotional resources for future social demands.

This pattern can create relationship difficulties when others interpret the need for post-social recovery as rejection or lack of interest in continued connection. Friends might feel confused when Jennifer seems enthusiastic during social events but then becomes unavailable for follow-up activities.

The invisible labor of emotional management

Daily life with quiet BPD involves tremendous amounts of invisible emotional labor—the ongoing work of regulating emotions, managing triggers, maintaining relationships, and monitoring internal and external states that others take for granted or handle automatically.

This emotional labor includes:

Trigger management: Constantly scanning environments and interactions for potential emotional triggers while developing strategies to avoid or manage them. This might involve planning routes to avoid certain locations, timing activities to minimize stress, or preparing emotionally for challenging situations.

Relationship maintenance: Monitoring multiple relationships for signs of problems, remembering important details about others' lives, and adjusting behavior to maintain connection and approval. This includes remembering birthdays, checking in with friends during difficult periods, and managing others' emotional needs.

Internal state monitoring: Tracking mood changes, physical symptoms, energy levels, and emotional reactions throughout the day. People with quiet BPD often develop sophisticated awareness of their internal states because small changes can signal the need for interventions or self-care.

Crisis prevention: Recognizing early warning signs of emotional overwhelm and implementing strategies to prevent crisis situations. This might involve taking breaks from social activities, adjusting work schedules, or seeking support before situations become unmanageable.

Identity maintenance: Working to maintain some sense of stable self while managing the pulls toward shapeshifting and people-pleasing. This includes regularly checking in with personal values, preferences, and goals to maintain some consistency across different social contexts.

Performance sustainability: Managing the energy required to maintain external functionality while dealing with internal emotional challenges. This includes pacing activities, building in recovery time, and making lifestyle adjustments that support emotional regulation.

Building sustainable daily routines

Recognition of quiet BPD's daily challenges creates opportunities to develop more sustainable routines that honor both internal emotional needs and external responsibilities. This involves finding ways to reduce decision fatigue, build in emotional recovery time, and create structure that supports emotional regulation.

Successful daily management strategies often include:

Decision simplification: Reducing the number of daily choices through routine establishment. This might involve planning weekly meal menus, creating standard clothing combinations, or developing go-to responses for common social situations.

Energy budgeting: Treating emotional energy as a finite resource that requires careful management. This includes scheduling demanding activities when energy levels are highest and building in recovery time after emotionally challenging events.

Authentic self check-ins: Regular times throughout the day to reconnect with genuine thoughts, feelings, and preferences. This might involve brief meditation, journaling, or simply asking yourself what you actually want or need in the moment.

Support system utilization: Developing relationships with people who understand quiet BPD challenges and can provide validation and support during difficult periods. This includes educating close friends and family about the condition and what kinds of support are most helpful.

Crisis planning: Preparing strategies for managing emotional overwhelm before crisis situations occur. This includes identifying early warning signs, developing self-soothing techniques, and knowing when to seek additional support.

Key understanding of daily quiet BPD experiences:

- Routine decisions become emotionally complex due to identity uncertainty, perfectionist analysis, and rejection sensitivity, creating decision paralysis around simple choices
- The chameleon effect involves constant self-monitoring and adjustment to match others' expectations, leading to exhaustion and identity confusion
- Emotional storms occur internally while maintaining external composure, creating invisible crises that others cannot recognize or support
- Social interactions require tremendous energy for emotional regulation and self-monitoring, necessitating recovery periods that others may misunderstand
- Daily life involves enormous amounts of invisible emotional labor including trigger management, relationship maintenance, and identity work
- Sustainable daily routines require decision simplification, energy budgeting, regular authenticity check-ins, and systematic crisis prevention planning
- Recognition of these daily challenges validates the real difficulties of living with quiet BPD while opening pathways toward more sustainable coping strategies

The next chapter will explore the journey of finding appropriate therapeutic help, examining how to identify effective treatments and navigate the unique challenges of therapy when your condition often remains invisible to mental health professionals.

Chapter 8: Finding the right help

The therapy journey that finally changed everything began with Dr. Patricia Williams asking an unusual question during their first session. Instead of inquiring about symptoms or family history, she asked Jennifer to describe how much energy it took to maintain her composed exterior during social interactions. "On a scale of one to ten," Dr. Williams said, "how exhausting is it to appear fine when you're struggling internally?"

Jennifer had never been asked this question in fifteen years of therapy attempts. Previous therapists had focused on her depression, anxiety, or relationship concerns without recognizing the tremendous effort required to function while managing intense internal emotional storms. Dr. Williams's question opened the door to understanding quiet BPD as more than just anxiety or depression—as a complex pattern of emotional regulation that required specialized therapeutic approaches.

This moment illustrates why finding effective help for quiet BPD often involves a lengthy search for clinicians who understand that high-functioning exterior presentations can mask significant internal distress and that traditional therapeutic approaches may not address the unique challenges of internalized emotional dysregulation.

The search for understanding

Jennifer's previous therapy experiences followed a familiar pattern for many people with quiet BPD. Well-meaning therapists provided accurate diagnoses for her secondary symptoms—depression, anxiety, perfectionism—without recognizing the underlying emotional dysregulation that drove these surface presentations. Each therapeutic relationship began hopefully and ended with Jennifer feeling understood but not fundamentally changed.

Dr. Sarah Martinez, Jennifer's third therapist, focused on cognitive-behavioral techniques for managing anxiety and depression. Jennifer learned valuable skills for challenging negative thoughts and managing panic attacks, but these interventions didn't address her core fears of abandonment or the identity instability that created ongoing relationship difficulties. Jennifer felt grateful for the practical skills but sensed that deeper patterns remained untouched.

Dr. Robert Chen, Jennifer's fifth therapist, provided insight-oriented therapy that helped Jennifer understand connections between her childhood experiences and current emotional patterns. These insights felt validating and intellectually satisfying, but Jennifer continued experiencing the same emotional intensity and relationship difficulties that had brought her to therapy initially. Understanding why she struggled didn't provide the emotional regulation skills needed to struggle less intensely.

The missing piece in Jennifer's treatment history was recognition that her high-functioning presentation masked borderline-level emotional dysregulation that required specialized interventions designed specifically for emotional regulation deficits rather than general anxiety or depression.

Why standard approaches fall short

Traditional therapeutic approaches often prove insufficient for quiet BPD because they weren't designed to address the specific combination of emotional intensity, identity instability, and internalized presentation that characterizes this condition. Several factors contribute to treatment effectiveness gaps:

Symptom focus vs. pattern recognition: Many therapeutic approaches target specific symptoms—anxiety, depression, perfectionism—rather than recognizing these as expressions of underlying emotional dysregulation patterns. Jennifer's anxiety wasn't generalized anxiety disorder requiring relaxation techniques; it was rejection sensitivity requiring different interventions focused on interpersonal effectiveness and distress tolerance.

Insight limitations: Understanding childhood origins of current difficulties provides valuable perspective but doesn't automatically translate into emotional regulation skills. Jennifer could clearly articulate how her parents' emotional unavailability contributed to her current relationship fears, but this insight didn't reduce the intensity of her emotional reactions when she perceived rejection.

Cognitive emphasis: Traditional cognitive-behavioral approaches emphasize changing thought patterns to influence emotions, but quiet BPD involves neurobiological differences in emotional processing that require more comprehensive interventions. Jennifer learned to challenge negative thoughts about herself and others, but the underlying emotional intensity persisted regardless of her cognitive efforts.

Individual focus: Many therapeutic approaches focus primarily on individual change without addressing the interpersonal dynamics that are central to BPD presentations. Jennifer's struggles occurred primarily in relationships, but her individual therapy sessions didn't provide opportunities to practice new interpersonal skills in real-time situations.

Functioning assumptions: Therapists often assume that high-functioning individuals have better emotional regulation skills and require less intensive interventions. Jennifer's external competence masked the need for specialized emotional regulation training that wasn't offered because she didn't appear to need it.

Dialectical behavior therapy adaptations

Dialectical Behavior Therapy (DBT) represents the gold-standard treatment for BPD, but standard DBT protocols were designed primarily for individuals with classic BPD presentations who struggle with external behavioral control. People with quiet BPD often need modifications to traditional DBT approaches because their challenges involve over-control rather than under-control of emotions and behaviors.

Dr. Williams explained to Jennifer that traditional DBT teaches skills for managing intense emotions that get expressed outwardly through self-harm, relationship chaos, or impulsive behaviors. Quiet BPD individuals need similar emotional regulation skills, but applied to internal rather than external emotional experiences.

Emotion regulation adaptations: Standard DBT emotion regulation skills focus on reducing emotional intensity and avoiding impulsive actions. For quiet BPD, the focus shifts to identifying and expressing emotions appropriately rather than suppressing them automatically. Jennifer learned to recognize when she was numbing emotions and practice allowing herself to feel without immediately trying to fix or change emotional experiences.

Distress tolerance modifications: Traditional DBT distress tolerance skills help people avoid destructive behaviors during emotional crises. Quiet BPD individuals need skills for tolerating emotional distress without engaging in internal self-punishment or complete emotional shutdown. Jennifer learned techniques for staying present during emotional difficulties without escaping into perfectionism or people-pleasing behaviors.

Interpersonal effectiveness adjustments: Standard DBT interpersonal skills focus on maintaining relationships while managing intense emotional expressions. Quiet BPD modifications emphasize expressing authentic needs and emotions in relationships rather than automatically prioritizing others' needs over your own. Jennifer practiced asking for support directly instead of hoping others would notice her indirect hints.

Mindfulness refinements: Traditional DBT mindfulness helps people observe their emotions without being overwhelmed by them. For quiet BPD, mindfulness practices focus on reconnecting with authentic emotional experiences that have been suppressed or dismissed. Jennifer learned to check in with her actual feelings and preferences throughout the day rather than automatically adapting to others' apparent expectations.

Radically Open DBT for the overcontrolled

Some individuals with quiet BPD benefit from Radically Open DBT (RO-DBT), a specialized approach developed specifically for people who over-control their emotions and behaviors rather than under-controlling them. RO-DBT recognizes that excessive emotional control can be just as problematic as insufficient control, requiring different therapeutic interventions.

Dr. Lynch, who developed RO-DBT, explains that overcontrolled individuals often possess excellent self-discipline and behavioral control but struggle with flexibility, emotional expression, and authentic social connections. These individuals appear highly functional but experience internal distress from suppressing natural emotional responses and maintaining rigid behavioral standards.

RO-DBT focuses on several key areas particularly relevant to quiet BPD:

Emotional expression training: Learning to express emotions appropriately rather than suppressing them automatically. This includes practicing vulnerable communication, sharing authentic feelings with trusted others, and tolerating the discomfort that emotional expression can initially create.

Flexible responding: Developing ability to adapt responses based on situational demands rather than maintaining rigid behavioral patterns. This might involve practicing saying no to requests, expressing different opinions, or allowing yourself to be imperfect in social situations.

Social connectedness: Building genuine relationships based on authenticity rather than performance. This includes learning to share personal struggles, accepting support from others, and developing friendships that can tolerate your complete emotional range.

Self-compassion development: Reducing harsh self-judgment and developing kindness toward yourself during difficult moments. This involves recognizing that perfectionism and self-criticism don't actually improve performance or prevent problems.

Schema therapy for healing early wounds

Schema Therapy provides another effective approach for quiet BPD by addressing the deep-seated emotional patterns that developed during childhood experiences of invalidation or neglect. Schema Therapy recognizes that current emotional difficulties often stem from adaptive responses to early life experiences that are no longer helpful in adult relationships.

Dr. Williams incorporated Schema Therapy concepts to help Jennifer understand how her current patterns connected to childhood experiences while developing new ways of responding to emotional triggers that didn't involve automatic self-suppression.

Schema identification: Jennifer learned to recognize her dominant schemas—core beliefs about herself and relationships that developed during childhood. Her "defectiveness" schema created persistent feelings of being fundamentally flawed, while her "emotional deprivation" schema generated expectations that others wouldn't be available to meet her emotional needs.

Schema triggers: Jennifer developed awareness of situations that activated her schemas, recognizing that current relationship events often triggered emotional responses that were disproportionate to the actual situation because they connected to historical emotional wounds.

Limited reparenting: Dr. Williams provided some of the emotional validation and support that Jennifer hadn't received during childhood, helping her develop internal resources for self-soothing and self-validation that she could access independently.

Schema healing: Jennifer learned techniques for responding to schema activation in ways that promoted healing rather than reinforcing old patterns. This included practicing self-compassion during moments of feeling defective and reaching out for support instead of automatically assuming others wouldn't be available.

The therapeutic relationship as healing agent

For individuals with quiet BPD, the therapeutic relationship itself often provides the most significant healing opportunity. Many people with quiet BPD have never experienced relationships where they could express authentic emotions without fear of rejection or criticism. The therapeutic relationship provides a safe laboratory for practicing vulnerability and emotional expression.

Dr. Williams's approach with Jennifer involved several relationship elements that proved particularly healing:

Consistent availability: Dr. Williams maintained reliable appointment times and consistent emotional presence during sessions, helping Jennifer experience what secure attachment feels like. This consistency helped Jennifer begin to trust that others could be dependable without her having to earn their reliability through perfect behavior.

Emotion validation: Dr. Williams consistently validated Jennifer's emotional experiences as understandable responses to her life circumstances rather than evidence of personal weakness or defectiveness. This validation helped Jennifer develop self-compassion and reduce the self-criticism that had been automatic for years.

Genuine curiosity: Rather than trying to fix Jennifer's problems quickly, Dr. Williams expressed authentic interest in understanding Jennifer's internal experience. This curiosity helped Jennifer become more curious about her own emotional patterns rather than judgmental about them.

Appropriate boundaries: Dr. Williams maintained professional boundaries while being emotionally available during sessions, helping Jennifer experience what healthy relationships look like. This boundary modeling helped Jennifer learn to maintain her own boundaries in other relationships.

Tolerance for emotional intensity: Dr. Williams didn't try to minimize or quickly resolve Jennifer's intense emotions, instead helping her learn to tolerate and explore these feelings. This tolerance helped Jennifer develop confidence that her emotional intensity wouldn't overwhelm others who cared about her.

Finding qualified therapists

Locating therapists qualified to treat quiet BPD requires research and persistence, as many mental health professionals haven't received specialized training in recognizing and treating internalized BPD presentations. Several strategies can improve your chances of finding effective help:

Training credentials: Look for therapists with specific training in BPD treatments like DBT, RO-DBT, Schema Therapy, or Mentalization-Based Treatment. These specialized approaches address emotional regulation and identity issues more directly than general therapy approaches.

Experience with high-functioning clients: Seek therapists who have experience working with individuals who appear functional externally but struggle with internal emotional regulation. Some therapists specialize in working with professionals, high achievers, or individuals with "invisible" mental health challenges.

Trauma-informed approaches: Many quiet BPD presentations involve histories of emotional neglect or invalidation that might not meet traditional trauma criteria but require trauma-informed therapeutic approaches. Look for therapists trained in complex trauma or developmental trauma.

Assessment capabilities: Effective therapists should be able to conduct comprehensive assessments that go beyond surface symptoms to identify underlying emotional regulation patterns and attachment styles. They should ask questions about your internal experience, not just your external behaviors.

Treatment planning: Qualified therapists should be able to explain how they'll address the specific challenges of quiet BPD, including emotional regulation skill-building, identity development, and relationship pattern changes. They should have concrete plans for addressing internalized rather than externalized symptoms.

Questions to ask potential therapists

When interviewing therapists, consider asking specific questions about their understanding and experience with quiet BPD:

- "How do you typically work with clients who appear high-functioning but struggle with internal emotional intensity?"
- "What experience do you have treating internalized or 'quiet' presentations of BPD?"
- "How would you approach emotional regulation difficulties in someone who over-controls rather than under-controls their emotions?"
- "What role does the therapeutic relationship play in your treatment approach?"
- "How do you help clients who struggle with identity instability and chronic feelings of emptiness?"

Their responses should demonstrate understanding that high-functioning presentations can mask significant internal distress and that specialized approaches may be needed for internalized emotional regulation difficulties.

Key understanding for finding effective quiet BPD treatment:

- Standard therapeutic approaches often fall short because they address surface symptoms rather than underlying emotional dysregulation patterns characteristic of quiet BPD
- Traditional DBT may need modifications for quiet BPD individuals who over-control rather than under-control their emotions and behaviors

- RO-DBT specifically addresses overcontrolled presentations and may be more appropriate for some quiet BPD individuals than standard DBT
- Schema Therapy effectively addresses childhood origins of current emotional patterns while building skills for responding differently to emotional triggers
- The therapeutic relationship itself provides crucial healing opportunities for individuals who haven't experienced safe emotional expression in relationships
- Finding qualified therapists requires research into specialized training and experience with high-functioning but internally struggling clients
- Asking specific questions about approaches to internalized emotional regulation can help identify therapists capable of providing effective quiet BPD treatment

The next chapter will explore how traditional DBT skills can be adapted and applied specifically for quiet BPD presentations, providing practical tools for managing internal emotional storms while maintaining external functionality.

Chapter 9: The DBT toolkit reimagined for quiet BPD

The conference room fell silent as Dr. Patricia Williams presented her findings to the clinical team. "Traditional DBT assumes emotional dysregulation manifests outwardly," she began, clicking to her next slide. "But what happens when a client already over-regulates their emotions? What happens when they need to learn to feel more, not less?" The room buzzed with recognition as clinicians considered their "model patients"—those articulate, compliant individuals who seemed to have excellent insight but never quite achieved lasting change.

This question represents a fundamental shift in how we approach DBT skills training for individuals with quiet BPD. The standard DBT model was designed for people who struggle with under-controlled emotions and behaviors—those who act impulsively, express anger dramatically, or engage in obvious self-destructive behaviors. Quiet BPD individuals present the opposite challenge: they over-control their emotions and behaviors to such an extent that they've become disconnected from their authentic emotional experiences.

Skills in action for the over-controlled mind

The DBT skills modules—mindfulness, emotion regulation, distress tolerance, and interpersonal effectiveness—require significant modifications when applied to quiet BPD presentations. Rather than learning to slow down emotional responses, these individuals need to learn to speed them up. Instead of containing behavioral impulses, they need permission to express authentic needs and feelings.

Consider Maria, a 31-year-old social worker who completed standard DBT skills training twice without significant improvement. Her therapists praised her excellent homework completion and skill implementation, yet Maria continued experiencing intense internal emotional storms while maintaining perfect external composure. The breakthrough came when her third therapist, trained in quiet BPD adaptations, asked a different question: "Maria, instead of using skills to contain your emotions, what would happen if you used them to explore what you're actually feeling?"

This shift from emotional containment to emotional exploration represents the core adaptation needed for quiet BPD applications. Traditional DBT teaches skills for managing overwhelming emotions; quiet BPD requires skills for accessing suppressed emotions and expressing them safely in relationships.

Emotion regulation when you're already over-regulating

Standard DBT emotion regulation focuses on reducing emotional intensity and duration. The assumption is that clients experience emotions too intensely for too long, creating problems in their daily functioning. Quiet BPD individuals often experience emotions with equal intensity but have learned to suppress, minimize, or intellectualize these feelings so effectively that they lose touch with their emotional guidance system.

The emotion identification challenge

Traditional DBT begins with emotion identification using basic feeling words and intensity scales. Quiet BPD clients can often identify emotions intellectually but struggle to connect with the bodily sensations and impulses that accompany feelings. They might say "I'm angry" while displaying no physical signs of anger and feeling no urge to address the situation that triggered the anger.

Lisa, a 35-year-old marketing executive, exemplifies this pattern. During DBT skills practice, she could accurately label her emotions and rate their intensity on a 1-10 scale. However, when asked to describe what anger felt like in her body or what it made her want to do, she would respond with blank confusion. Lisa had learned to recognize emotions intellectually without allowing herself to experience them physically or behaviorally.

The adapted approach involves **somatic emotion exploration**—learning to notice the subtle physical sensations that accompany emotions before they get intellectualized or suppressed. Lisa practiced the "body scan for emotions" technique, slowly moving her attention through her body while recalling recent interactions, looking for areas of tension, warmth, or other sensations that might indicate emotional responses.

Modified emotional experiencing exercises

Rather than using traditional emotion regulation skills to reduce emotional intensity, quiet BPD clients need exercises that increase their capacity to tolerate and explore emotional experiences. The **"emotion amplification technique"** involves deliberately focusing on emotional experiences to understand their full message and meaning.

During a session, Lisa recalled a workplace interaction where her supervisor had criticized her project approach. Using traditional DBT, she would have used distraction or opposite action to reduce the emotional impact. Instead, she practiced amplifying the emotional experience: sitting quietly, breathing into the feeling, and allowing herself to fully experience her anger without immediately trying to rationalize or minimize it.

This practice revealed information that Lisa's quick emotional suppression had been hiding: her anger contained important messages about boundary violations, unmet needs for recognition, and her pattern of accepting criticism too readily. The anger wasn't a problem to be regulated—it was emotional data that could guide her toward healthier workplace interactions.

Opposite action modifications

Traditional DBT's opposite action skill teaches clients to act opposite to their emotional urges when emotions are unjustified or ineffective. For quiet BPD, the modification focuses on acting opposite to their **suppression urges** rather than their emotional urges. The skill becomes: "When you have the urge to suppress, minimize, or intellectualize an emotion, act opposite by expressing, amplifying, or physically experiencing it."

James, a 29-year-old teacher, used modified opposite action when he felt hurt by a friend's cancellation of their dinner plans. His automatic response was to tell himself it didn't matter, make excuses for his friend, and suppress his disappointment. Using opposite action for suppression, James instead allowed himself to feel disappointed, acknowledged that the cancellation did affect him, and chose to express his feelings to his friend rather than pretending everything was fine.

Distress tolerance for internal crises

Traditional distress tolerance skills help clients survive crisis situations without making them worse through impulsive actions. Quiet BPD individuals rarely engage in external crisis behaviors, but they experience intense internal crises that can be equally destabilizing. Their distress tolerance skills need to focus on surviving internal emotional storms without engaging in self-attack, emotional numbing, or other internal escape behaviors.

The internal crisis experience

Rebecca, a 33-year-old nurse, describes her internal crises as "emotional earthquakes that no one else can see." During a typical episode, triggered by a perceived criticism from a colleague, Rebecca would experience racing thoughts, physical anxiety symptoms, and overwhelming shame while continuing to perform her nursing duties normally. Her colleagues saw a competent professional; she experienced emotional chaos.

Traditional distress tolerance skills like ice water or intense exercise didn't address Rebecca's specific challenge. Her crisis wasn't about preventing external behaviors—it was about surviving internal emotional intensity without engaging in self-punishment or complete emotional shutdown.

Modified distress tolerance techniques

The **"internal grounding"** technique helps quiet BPD individuals stay present during internal emotional storms without appearing distressed to others. This involves subtle grounding practices that can be used in social or professional situations: pressing feet firmly into the floor, secretly counting objects in the environment, or using discrete breathing patterns.

Rebecca learned to use the "5-4-3-2-1 grounding technique" modified for workplace use. During emotional storms, she would mentally identify five things she could see, four things she could hear, three things she could touch, two things she could smell, and one thing she could taste, all while maintaining normal work activities. This grounding prevented her from spiraling into complete internal chaos while remaining invisible to colleagues.

The **"self-compassion in crisis"** skill addresses the tendency for quiet BPD individuals to engage in harsh self-criticism during emotional difficulties. Instead of traditional distraction techniques, this skill involves offering yourself the same compassion you would offer a good friend experiencing similar difficulties.

When Rebecca noticed herself beginning the familiar self-attack patterns ("You're overreacting," "You're too sensitive," "Everyone else can handle this"), she would practice the self-compassion script: "This is a moment of suffering. Suffering is part of human experience. May I be kind to myself during this difficult time."

Crisis urge surfing

While traditional DBT teaches urge surfing for behavioral impulses, quiet BPD individuals need skills for surfing their urges to engage in internal escape behaviors. The most common internal escape urges include: numbing emotions through overthinking, engaging in self-punishment thoughts, or completely shutting down emotionally.

Marcus, a 27-year-old graphic designer, learned to recognize his urges to "escape" into work perfectionism whenever he felt emotional pain. Instead of giving in to these urges, he practiced "urge surfing"—

observing the urge to escape without acting on it, while allowing the underlying emotional pain to exist without immediately trying to fix or escape it.

Interpersonal effectiveness for conflict-avoiders

Traditional DBT interpersonal effectiveness focuses on getting needs met while maintaining relationships and self-respect. For quiet BPD individuals, the primary challenge isn't maintaining relationships— they're often exceptional at preserving relationships through people-pleasing and conflict avoidance. Their challenge is learning to express authentic needs and emotions in relationships without losing the other person's approval.

The authentic expression challenge

Traditional DBT assumes clients know what they want and need but struggle with how to ask for it effectively. Quiet BPD clients often struggle with knowing what they actually want and need because they've spent years prioritizing others' needs over their own. Before they can use interpersonal effectiveness skills, they need skills for identifying their authentic preferences and needs.

Amanda, a 26-year-old veterinarian, could use DEAR MAN (Describe, Express, Assert, Reinforce, Mindful, Appear confident, Negotiate) techniques perfectly in role-plays but struggled to identify what she wanted to ask for in her real relationships. Her automatic response in conflicts was to find out what the other person wanted and then try to provide it, even when this meant ignoring her own needs.

Modified needs identification process

The **"authentic wants inventory"** helps quiet BPD individuals reconnect with their genuine preferences and needs. This involves regular check-ins throughout the day asking: "What do I actually want right now?" and "What do I need in this situation?" without immediately considering what's realistic or what others might prefer.

Amanda practiced this inventory during routine interactions: "What do I want for dinner?" "What do I need from this conversation?" "How do I want to spend my evening?" Initially, she often answered "I don't know" or immediately defaulted to what seemed appropriate. With practice, she began recognizing subtle preferences and needs that she had been automatically suppressing.

Conflict engagement skills

While traditional DBT focuses on managing conflict effectively, quiet BPD modifications focus on **entering** conflict when it's necessary for relationship health. This involves skills for recognizing when conflict avoidance is harming relationships and finding ways to address differences directly while managing the anxiety that conflict triggers.

The **"gentle confrontation"** technique teaches quiet BPD individuals to address relationship issues directly but in ways that feel emotionally safe. This involves using "I" statements about your experience rather than "you" statements about the other person's behavior, focusing on specific situations rather than character issues, and expressing your needs clearly while remaining open to compromise.

When Amanda's roommate consistently left dishes unwashed, her traditional response was to clean them herself while building internal resentment. Using gentle confrontation, she said: "I feel stressed when I come home to dishes in the sink because I need our shared spaces to feel clean and organized. Could we work out a system that works for both of us?"

Mindfulness for the chronically disconnected

Traditional DBT mindfulness helps clients observe their experiences without being overwhelmed by them. Quiet BPD individuals often observe their experiences too much—analyzing, intellectualizing, and evaluating their emotions and reactions constantly. They need mindfulness skills that help them **participate** in their emotional experiences rather than just observing them from a distance.

The over-thinking trap

Kevin, a 32-year-old accountant, exemplified the quiet BPD relationship with mindfulness. He could observe his emotions with remarkable clarity, describing their triggers, physical sensations, and patterns with therapeutic precision. However, this observation often became another form of emotional distancing—he would analyze his feelings rather than feeling them.

Traditional "observe" skills encouraged Kevin to step back from his emotions and notice them objectively. This approach actually worsened his disconnection because stepping back from emotions was already his default coping mechanism. He needed mindfulness skills that brought him closer to his emotional experiences, not further away.

Participatory mindfulness techniques

The **"emotion embodiment"** practice teaches quiet BPD individuals to participate fully in their emotional experiences rather than observing them analytically. This involves deliberately focusing on the physical sensations of emotions, allowing them to move through your body, and staying present with the experience without immediately trying to understand or categorize it.

Kevin practiced emotion embodiment during his weekly therapy sessions. When discussing difficult relationship situations, instead of immediately analyzing his reactions, he would pause and ask: "What is this feeling like in my body right now?" He would then spend several minutes breathing into the physical sensations of the emotion, allowing himself to experience it fully before discussing what it might mean or how to respond to it.

Present moment re-engagement

Quiet BPD individuals often live primarily in their heads, analyzing past interactions and anticipating future problems. The **"sensory anchoring"** technique helps them return to present moment experience through deliberate attention to physical sensations.

Throughout his day, Kevin would practice "sensory check-ins": deliberately noticing five physical sensations he was experiencing in the current moment. This might include the feeling of his feet in his shoes, the temperature of the air on his skin, the taste in his mouth, the sounds in his environment, and the sensation of his breathing. These anchors helped bring him out of analytical thinking and into present moment experience.

Practice exercises and modified worksheets

The following adaptations transform standard DBT worksheets for quiet BPD applications:

Modified Emotion Regulation Worksheet

Instead of tracking emotional triggers and intensity, quiet BPD individuals track:

- Situations where you suppressed or minimized emotions
- Physical sensations you ignored or dismissed
- Times you intellectualized feelings rather than experiencing them
- Moments when you prioritized others' emotional needs over your own

Adapted Distress Tolerance Planning

Rather than planning for behavioral crises, create plans for:

- Internal emotional storms (shame spirals, anxiety attacks, identity confusion)
- Self-compassion strategies for moments of self-criticism
- Grounding techniques that work in social/professional settings
- Ways to reach out for support when you appear fine externally

Interpersonal Effectiveness for Authenticity

Modified DEAR MAN includes:

- **Detect**: Identify what you actually want or need (not what seems appropriate)
- **Express**: Share your authentic thoughts and feelings
- **Assert**: Ask directly for what you need
- **Reinforce**: Explain why your request matters to you
- **Mindful**: Stay present with your needs during the interaction
- **Appear**: Show up as your authentic self, not your people-pleasing persona
- **Negotiate**: Find solutions that honor both people's needs

Mindfulness for Connection

Instead of traditional observe-describe-participate, use:

- **Connect**: Tune into your body and physical experience
- **Allow**: Let emotions exist without immediately analyzing them
- **Engage**: Participate fully in the current moment experience

Putting it all together

Sarah, a 38-year-old attorney, spent six months learning these modified DBT skills after years of traditional therapy that hadn't addressed her core patterns. Her breakthrough moment came during a partner meeting at her law firm when a colleague criticized her case strategy.

Using traditional skills, Sarah would have observed her anger, analyzed why it felt so intense, and used opposite action to respond professionally while suppressing her emotional reaction. Instead, she used the quiet BPD adaptations:

1. **Connected** with her physical experience of anger rather than immediately intellectualizing it
2. **Allowed** herself to feel angry without immediately judging the emotion as inappropriate
3. **Identified** what she needed in the situation (acknowledgment of her expertise and respectful feedback)

4. **Expressed** her perspective using gentle confrontation: "I feel concerned when my approach is characterized as inadequate because I've researched this strategy thoroughly. I'd appreciate feedback that acknowledges the thought I've put into this."

This response honored both her authentic emotional experience and the professional relationship, demonstrating how modified DBT skills can help quiet BPD individuals express themselves authentically while maintaining appropriate boundaries.

Clinical wisdom for practitioners

The most effective DBT modifications for quiet BPD require therapists to reverse many traditional assumptions about emotional regulation. Instead of helping clients contain overwhelming emotions, we help them access suppressed emotions. Instead of reducing emotional intensity, we increase their capacity to tolerate authentic feeling. Instead of maintaining behavioral control, we encourage appropriate emotional expression.

This reversal can feel counterintuitive for therapists trained in traditional DBT approaches. The key is recognizing that emotional over-control can be just as problematic as emotional under-control, requiring different interventions that address the specific challenges of internalized emotional dysregulation.

The modified skills work best when combined with therapeutic relationships that model emotional authenticity and acceptance. Clients need to experience what it feels like to express genuine emotions without losing important relationships, starting with the safety of the therapeutic relationship and gradually extending these skills to other important connections in their lives.

Practical takeaways

- Traditional DBT skills require significant modifications for quiet BPD because these individuals over-control rather than under-control their emotions

- Emotion regulation adaptations focus on accessing and amplifying emotions rather than containing them
- Distress tolerance skills address internal crises and self-attack patterns rather than external behavioral impulses
- Interpersonal effectiveness modifications emphasize authentic expression and conflict engagement rather than relationship maintenance
- Mindfulness practices encourage emotional participation rather than analytical observation
- Modified worksheets track emotional suppression, internal experiences, and authenticity rather than external behaviors
- Success requires therapeutic relationships that model emotional safety and acceptance of authentic expression

Chapter 10: Beyond therapy: Holistic healing approaches

The turning point in Dr. Elena Rodriguez's recovery came not in a traditional therapy session, but during her first EMDR session when she processed a seemingly minor childhood memory. As a 12-year-old, she had excitedly shared her science fair project with her father, only to watch his face shift from interest to distraction as he answered his phone mid-sentence. The memory had seemed insignificant compared to obvious traumas, yet processing it through EMDR revealed layers of emotional suppression, people-pleasing patterns, and the deep-seated belief that her enthusiasm was too much for others to handle.

This experience illustrates why quiet BPD often requires healing approaches that extend beyond traditional talk therapy. The subtle emotional wounds that contribute to internalized borderline patterns may not respond to purely cognitive interventions, requiring treatments that access the body's wisdom, creative expression, and the nervous system's capacity for healing.

EMDR for processing hidden trauma

Eye Movement Desensitization and Reprocessing (EMDR) has proven particularly effective for quiet BPD because it addresses the subtle traumatic experiences that traditional trauma-focused therapies might overlook. Many individuals with quiet BPD carry what therapists call "small-t traumas"—experiences that weren't dramatically abusive but were emotionally invalidating enough to shape core beliefs about self-worth and relationships.

Understanding developmental trauma in quiet BPD

Dr. Martinez, Elena's EMDR therapist, explains that quiet BPD often develops from what she calls "death by a thousand paper cuts"—countless small experiences of emotional invalidation that accumulate into significant psychological wounds. These experiences might include:

- Parents who consistently responded to emotional expressions with mild annoyance or distraction
- Family systems that valued achievement and composure over emotional authenticity
- Childhood environments where sensitivity was treated as a problem to be fixed
- School or social experiences where emotional intensity resulted in rejection or criticism

Traditional therapy approaches might identify these patterns intellectually, but EMDR allows the nervous system to process and integrate these experiences at a somatic level, often resulting in profound shifts in emotional regulation and self-perception.

The EMDR process adapted for quiet BPD

Elena's EMDR treatment followed a modified protocol that accounted for her tendency to intellectualize rather than feel her emotional experiences. Her therapist used several adaptations:

Extended preparation phase: Traditional EMDR preparation focuses on developing coping skills for managing intense emotions during processing. Elena's preparation emphasized skills for **allowing** emotions rather than managing them, including somatic awareness techniques and practices for tolerating emotional intensity without immediately trying to understand or fix it.

Body-focused targeting: Instead of focusing solely on disturbing images or thoughts, Elena's therapist helped her identify where emotional memories were stored in her body. The phone call memory was "held" as tension in her chest and a collapsing sensation in her shoulders—physical memories of deflation and self-containment that had become automatic responses to emotional disappointment.

Gentle titration: Because Elena had spent years suppressing emotional responses, her nervous system needed careful titration during processing. Her therapist would pause frequently to help Elena track her physical responses, ensuring she remained present and connected to her body throughout the process rather than dissociating or intellectualizing.

Integration of positive beliefs: Traditional EMDR focuses on installing positive beliefs after processing negative memories. Elena's protocol emphasized installing beliefs about emotional authenticity and self-expression: "My emotions are acceptable," "I can be enthusiastic without being too much," and "Others can handle my emotional intensity."

After six months of EMDR processing, Elena reported significant changes in her daily emotional experience. She no longer felt compelled to edit her responses before sharing them with others, could express disappointment directly rather than through passive withdrawal, and experienced emotions as information rather than problems requiring immediate solutions.

Case example: Processing emotional invalidation

Marcus, a 34-year-old engineer, used EMDR to process what he initially dismissed as a "stupid memory" from high school. During a family dinner, he had shared his excitement about being accepted to engineering school, only to have his mother respond with concerns about the difficulty and competitiveness of the field. The memory hadn't felt traumatic at the time—his mother was trying to be helpful—but it captured a lifelong pattern of his enthusiasm being met with caution and concern.

EMDR processing revealed how this pattern had shaped his adult relationships. Marcus had learned to present his achievements and interests with disclaimers and downplay his excitement to prevent others from worrying or offering unsolicited advice. He realized he had been protecting others from his emotional intensity while depriving himself of the joy that comes from sharing positive experiences authentically.

Processing this memory through EMDR allowed Marcus to separate his mother's anxiety from his own experience of success. He developed the ability to receive others' concerns without automatically adopting them as his own, and learned to share positive experiences with appropriate enthusiasm rather than pre-emptive apologies.

Medication realities for quiet BPD

The relationship between quiet BPD and psychotropic medications is complex and often frustrating for both individuals and prescribing clinicians. Unlike conditions such as major depression or anxiety disorders, BPD represents a pattern of emotional dysregulation and identity disturbance that doesn't typically respond to medication as a primary treatment. However, many individuals with quiet BPD do benefit from medications that address co-occurring conditions or support their overall emotional regulation.

The medication myth and reality

Dr. Jennifer Liu, a psychiatrist specializing in personality disorders, addresses common misconceptions about medication and quiet BPD: "There's no medication for BPD itself, but that doesn't mean medication can't be helpful. The key is understanding what we're treating—are we addressing BPD symptoms directly, or are we supporting emotional regulation so that therapy can be more effective?"

Many individuals with quiet BPD carry shame about medication use, feeling that needing pharmaceutical support indicates personal failure or weakness. This shame often stems from their perfectionistic tendencies and the social messaging that suggests emotional difficulties should be resolved through willpower and self-improvement alone.

Medications that may help with co-occurring conditions

Research indicates that approximately 85% of individuals with BPD meet criteria for at least one other mental health condition, making medication management complex and individualized. For quiet BPD, the most commonly helpful medications include:

Antidepressants for mood stabilization: While antidepressants don't treat BPD directly, they can help stabilize mood baseline sufficiently for individuals to engage more effectively in therapy. Sarah, a 29-year-old teacher, found that a low dose of sertraline reduced her daily emotional volatility enough that she could practice new interpersonal skills without being overwhelmed by emotional intensity.

Anti-anxiety medications for specific situations: Short-term anti-anxiety medications can help quiet BPD individuals navigate specific challenging situations—job interviews, social events, or family gatherings—that might otherwise trigger overwhelming emotional responses. The key is using these medications strategically rather than as daily emotional avoidance tools.

Sleep medications for regulation support: Quality sleep is fundamental to emotional regulation, and many individuals with quiet BPD struggle with insomnia related to rumination and anxiety. Sleep medications used temporarily can establish healthy sleep patterns that support overall emotional stability.

Mood stabilizers for emotional intensity: Some individuals benefit from mood stabilizing medications that help reduce the intensity of emotional swings without numbing emotional experiences entirely. These medications work best when combined with therapy that helps individuals develop skills for working with their emotions rather than simply containing them.

Group therapy for finding your voice

Group therapy presents unique challenges and opportunities for individuals with quiet BPD. Their tendency toward people-pleasing and emotional suppression can initially make group participation feel safer than individual therapy, but it can also prevent them from accessing the full benefits of group healing. However, when facilitated appropriately, group therapy provides irreplaceable opportunities for practicing authentic expression and receiving feedback about their interpersonal patterns.

The group therapy paradox

Traditional group therapy assumes that members will naturally express their thoughts and feelings as part of the therapeutic process. Quiet BPD individuals often excel at appearing engaged and therapeutic without revealing their authentic emotional experiences. They become the "perfect group members"—supportive of others, insightful about interpersonal dynamics, and cooperative with group processes—while remaining essentially invisible as individuals with their own healing needs.

Dr. Rebecca Thompson runs specialized groups for high-functioning individuals with emotional regulation challenges. She explains the paradox: "These group members will give beautiful, therapeutic responses to others' shares, demonstrate excellent empathy and insight, and appear to be getting tremendous benefit from the group. Then you realize they haven't shared anything genuinely vulnerable about their own experience in six months of group participation."

Modified group therapy approaches

Process groups with authentic expression requirements: Some groups establish norms that require members to share at least one authentic emotional experience per session. This structure prevents quiet BPD members from hiding in their helper role while creating safe opportunities for practicing vulnerability.

Lisa joined a process group after individual therapy had helped her recognize her emotional patterns but hadn't given her opportunities to practice new ways of relating. The group's structure required each member to check in with their current emotional state and share one challenge they were currently facing. Initially terrifying for Lisa, this structure gradually taught her that others could handle her emotional intensity and that relationships could deepen through authentic sharing rather than perfect support-giving.

Skills-based groups with interpersonal practice: DBT groups specifically modified for quiet BPD focus heavily on interpersonal effectiveness practice. Members practice expressing disagreement, asking for support, and setting boundaries within the group setting, receiving immediate feedback about their interpersonal impact.

Therapeutic community approaches: Some treatment programs use therapeutic community models where quiet BPD individuals live in structured environments that require authentic emotional participation. These intensive programs can break through the isolation and emotional suppression that outpatient therapy might not adequately address.

Case example: Group breakthrough

Jennifer had attended a weekly process group for eight months, regularly offering thoughtful support to other members while sharing only surface-level personal experiences. Her breakthrough came during a group session when another member gently confronted her: "Jennifer, you always have such wise things to say about everyone else's problems, but I realize I don't know anything about what's actually hard for you."

This feedback initially triggered Jennifer's familiar shame response—she had been "caught" being inauthentic and felt exposed as a fraud. However, the group's supportive response to her shame surprised her. Instead of rejection or criticism, other members shared their appreciation for her support while expressing genuine curiosity about her inner experience. This moment taught Jennifer that others actually wanted to know her authentic self, not just her helpful persona.

Over the following months, Jennifer gradually learned to share her own struggles with perfectionism, relationship anxiety, and fear of being too much for others. The group became a laboratory for practicing emotional authenticity, teaching her that relationships could become deeper and more satisfying when she brought her genuine self to them.

Body-based approaches for emotional reconnection

Many individuals with quiet BPD have become so skilled at emotional suppression that they've lost connection with their body's emotional wisdom. Traditional talk therapies work primarily with cognitive and verbal processing, but emotional healing often requires accessing the somatic experiences where feelings are stored and expressed.

The body-mind connection in quiet BPD

Trauma specialist Dr. Michael Chen explains how emotional suppression affects the body: "When we consistently suppress emotional expression, we're not just managing our minds—we're training our bodies to hold emotional energy without releasing it. Over time, this creates patterns of chronic tension, disconnection, and physical symptoms that talk therapy alone may not address."

Individuals with quiet BPD often report:

- Chronic muscle tension, particularly in the neck, shoulders, and jaw
- Digestive issues related to stress and emotional suppression
- Sleep difficulties stemming from inability to "turn off" mental activity
- Physical numbness or disconnection from bodily sensations
- Fatigue from the energy required to maintain emotional control

Somatic experiencing and emotional release

Somatic Experiencing (SE) helps individuals reconnect with their body's natural capacity for emotional regulation and release. This approach recognizes that trauma and chronic emotional suppression are stored in the nervous system and require body-based interventions for complete healing.

Rachel worked with a somatic experiencing practitioner after years of traditional therapy had helped her understand her patterns intellectually without creating significant emotional change. Her SE sessions involved learning to track physical sensations, notice areas of tension or numbness, and allow her body's natural healing responses to emerge.

During one session, while discussing a recent conflict with her partner, Rachel noticed tension building in her chest and shoulders. Instead of immediately talking about the conflict, her practitioner encouraged her to breathe into the sensation and notice what her body wanted to do. Rachel discovered an impulse to push away with her hands—a physical expression of the boundary she had been unable to set verbally. Practicing this physical movement while discussing the conflict helped Rachel access both the emotional clarity and physical empowerment needed to address the relationship issue directly.

Yoga and movement therapy adaptations

Traditional yoga practices require modifications for individuals with quiet BPD because their tendency toward perfectionism and self-criticism can turn even healing practices into another area for self-judgment. Trauma-informed yoga approaches emphasize choice, body awareness, and emotional safety over physical achievement.

Breath work for emotional regulation: Specific breathing practices can help quiet BPD individuals develop capacity for tolerating emotional intensity while remaining present in their bodies. Box breathing, alternate nostril breathing, and other techniques provide concrete tools for managing emotional storms without completely suppressing them.

Mindful movement for reconnection: Dance/movement therapy and other expressive movement practices help individuals reconnect with emotional impulses that have been suppressed. These approaches work particularly well for people who have difficulty accessing emotions through talking alone.

Creative therapies for authentic expression

Art, music, and creative expression provide alternative pathways for accessing and expressing the emotions that quiet BPD individuals have learned to suppress verbally. Creative therapies bypass some of the intellectual defenses and people-pleasing patterns that can interfere with traditional talk therapy.

Art therapy for emotional exploration

Dr. Sandra Martinez, an art therapist specializing in personality disorders, explains why creative expression works particularly well for quiet BPD: "These individuals have often learned that their emotional expressions need to be appropriate, understandable, and contained. Art allows them to express emotional experiences that don't fit into neat verbal categories."

David had struggled in traditional therapy to identify and express his emotional experiences. His art therapy sessions provided a different avenue for emotional exploration. His paintings revealed emotional themes that he hadn't been able to articulate verbally—sense of being trapped behind glass, feelings of invisibility, and intense longing for connection that felt too vulnerable to express directly.

The art became a bridge between his internal emotional world and verbal processing. Looking at his paintings, David could identify feelings and patterns that had remained invisible when he tried to access them through talking alone. The visual representations of his emotional experience became reference points for deeper therapeutic work.

Music therapy for emotional expression

Music therapy provides both receptive experiences (listening to music) and active experiences (creating music) that can facilitate emotional processing. For quiet BPD individuals, music often provides a safe container for experiencing emotional intensity that feels overwhelming in other contexts.

Playlist therapy: Creating playlists that represent different emotional states helps individuals develop more nuanced emotional vocabulary and provides tools for emotional regulation. Sarah created different playlists for various emotional states—anger, sadness, anxiety, joy—and used them both to process difficult emotions and to practice tolerating emotional intensity.

Instrument-based expression: Learning to play instruments provides a physical outlet for emotional expression that doesn't require verbal articulation. The rhythm, volume, and intensity of musical expression can mirror emotional experiences in ways that words sometimes cannot capture.

Building your personal healing toolkit

Recovery from quiet BPD typically requires a combination of approaches rather than relying on any single therapeutic modality. The most effective healing plans include elements that address cognitive patterns, emotional regulation, somatic healing, and interpersonal skill development.

Assessment for holistic treatment planning

The first step in building a comprehensive healing approach involves honest assessment of which areas need attention:

Cognitive patterns: Do you struggle with perfectionist thinking, harsh self-criticism, or all-or-nothing beliefs about yourself and relationships?

Emotional regulation: Are you over-controlling emotions (suppressing and minimizing) or under-controlling them (feeling overwhelmed and reactive)?

Somatic connection: Do you feel connected to your body's signals, or have you learned to ignore physical sensations and needs?

Interpersonal skills: Can you express authentic needs and feelings in relationships, or do you default to people-pleasing and conflict avoidance?

Trauma processing: Do you carry emotional wounds from childhood invalidation, neglect, or other experiences that continue to influence your current relationships?

Integration and self-advocacy

The most challenging aspect of holistic healing involves advocating for the combination of treatments you need while managing the practical realities of insurance coverage, provider availability, and time constraints. Many individuals benefit from working with a primary therapist who can help coordinate different treatment modalities and ensure that various approaches support rather than conflict with each other.

Building a personal healing toolkit requires patience and experimentation. What works for one person with quiet BPD may not work for another, and treatment needs often change as healing progresses. The goal isn't to find the perfect combination immediately, but to remain open to different approaches while maintaining focus on the core goals of emotional authenticity, relationship satisfaction, and sustainable self-care.

Reflections on healing

The journey beyond traditional therapy requires courage to explore healing modalities that may feel unfamiliar or challenging. For individuals with quiet BPD, this exploration often involves learning to trust their body's wisdom, express emotions creatively, and allow others to witness their authentic emotional experiences. The approaches described in this chapter provide pathways for accessing the parts of healing that words alone cannot reach, supporting the deep emotional integration that lasting recovery requires.

- EMDR effectively processes the subtle emotional invalidation experiences that contribute to quiet BPD development
- Medication can support emotional regulation and co-occurring conditions but doesn't treat BPD directly
- Group therapy provides irreplaceable opportunities for practicing authentic expression with immediate interpersonal feedback
- Body-based therapies address the somatic effects of chronic emotional suppression that talk therapy alone may not reach
- Creative therapies bypass intellectual defenses and provide alternative pathways for emotional expression and exploration
- Holistic healing requires individualized combinations of treatment approaches rather than relying on any single therapeutic modality
- Building a comprehensive healing toolkit requires patience, experimentation, and advocacy for the services that support your unique recovery needs

Chapter 11: Communication and connection

The weekly family dinner at the Morrison household followed the same predictable pattern for twenty-three years. Polite conversation about work and weather, careful avoidance of anything emotionally charged, and Sarah's familiar role as the family diplomat—smoothing over tensions, redirecting uncomfortable topics, and ensuring everyone felt comfortable. What looked like family harmony from the outside was actually an elaborate emotional choreography designed to prevent anyone from experiencing discomfort or conflict.

Sarah's breakthrough came during her fourth year of therapy when she realized that her family's "close relationships" were actually built on mutual emotional suppression rather than genuine intimacy. Learning to speak her truth—to express authentic thoughts and feelings rather than manufactured pleasantness—required dismantling decades of communication patterns that had seemed loving but were actually preventing real connection.

This transformation from withdrawal to expression represents one of the most challenging aspects of quiet BPD recovery. Breaking the silence means risking the rejection and abandonment that emotional suppression was designed to prevent, yet it's the only pathway toward the authentic relationships that make life meaningful.

From withdrawal to expression

The journey from emotional withdrawal to authentic expression requires understanding the difference between healthy communication and the performed communication that many individuals with quiet BPD have perfected. Healthy communication includes the full range of human emotional experience—disagreement, disappointment, excitement, anger, joy, and vulnerability. Performed communication carefully edits emotional experiences to maintain others' comfort and approval.

Understanding communication patterns in quiet BPD

Dr. Amanda Richardson, a communication specialist who works with personality disorders, identifies several patterns that characterize quiet BPD communication:

Emotional editing: Automatically filtering thoughts and feelings before expressing them, removing anything that might cause discomfort or conflict. Sarah had become so skilled at this editing that she often forgot what she actually thought or felt about situations by the time she finished crafting her "appropriate" response.

Preemptive apologizing: Beginning conversations with apologies for sharing, speaking, or potentially inconveniencing others. This pattern communicates that your thoughts and feelings are burdensome before you've even expressed them.

Opinion morphing: Automatically adjusting your expressed opinions to match what others seem to want to hear. This happens so subtly that individuals often don't recognize they're doing it, instead genuinely believing they agree with others more than they actually do.

Emotional minimization: Consistently downplaying the intensity or importance of your emotional experiences when communicating with others. "I'm a little disappointed" when you're devastated, or "It's not a big deal" when something is very important to you.

Indirect expression: Communicating needs and feelings through hints, implications, and subtle cues rather than direct statements. This allows for plausible deniability if the other person doesn't respond positively—you can pretend you weren't really asking for anything.

Learning to speak your truth

The process of developing authentic communication begins with reconnecting with your actual thoughts and feelings before attempting to share them with others. Many individuals with quiet BPD have become so disconnected from their authentic responses that they need to rebuild the capacity to know what they think and feel before they can express it.

Authentic response identification

Before Sarah could learn to communicate authentically, she needed to learn to recognize her authentic responses to situations. This required developing what her therapist called "emotional curiosity"—the practice of checking in with herself to discover what she was actually experiencing rather than what she thought she should be experiencing.

The process involved regular self-inquiry throughout the day:

- What am I actually feeling about this situation?
- What do I genuinely think about what just happened?
- What do I want or need right now?
- How do I really want to respond to this person?

Initially, Sarah's answers were often "I don't know" because she had spent years automatically suppressing her authentic responses in favor of socially appropriate ones. Learning to tolerate not knowing while staying curious about her internal experience gradually helped her reconnect with feelings and opinions that had been buried under layers of people-pleasing.

Case example: The workplace disagreement

Michael's transformation in authentic expression began with a seemingly minor workplace disagreement. During a team meeting, his supervisor proposed a project approach that Michael believed was inefficient and likely to create problems later. His traditional response would have been to find diplomatic ways to support the supervisor's idea while privately worrying about the potential consequences.

Using his new authentic communication skills, Michael practiced identifying his genuine response: he felt concerned about the proposed approach and believed his alternative suggestion would be more effective. He also identified his fears about expressing disagreement: that his supervisor might view him as difficult or uncooperative.

Instead of letting his fears prevent him from speaking, Michael used a direct but respectful approach: "I have some concerns about this approach and would like to suggest an alternative. I'm worried that the timeline we're discussing might create quality issues, and I think we could address those concerns by adjusting our sequence of tasks."

The supervisor's positive response surprised Michael—rather than viewing his input as problematic, she appreciated his thoughtful analysis and incorporated his suggestions into the project plan. This experience taught Michael that his authentic professional input was valuable and that expressing genuine concerns could strengthen rather than damage workplace relationships.

Validation techniques for self and others

Validation—the act of acknowledging and accepting emotional experiences as understandable—represents a core skill for building authentic relationships. Individuals with quiet BPD often struggle with both self-validation (accepting their own emotions as reasonable) and validating others appropriately (without automatically adopting others' emotions as their own).

Self-validation skills

Traditional validation teaches individuals to seek understanding and acceptance from others, but quiet BPD recovery requires developing internal validation skills that don't depend on others' responses. Self-validation means acknowledging your emotional experiences as reasonable given your circumstances, history, and current situation.

The internal validation process involves several steps:

1. **Recognition**: Notice when you're experiencing an emotion without immediately judging it as appropriate or inappropriate

2. **Acknowledgment**: Accept that you're having this emotional response without trying to change it immediately
3. **Understanding**: Explore what circumstances or triggers contributed to this emotional response
4. **Normalization**: Recognize that this emotional response makes sense given your situation
5. **Self-compassion**: Treat yourself with kindness during difficult emotional experiences

Jennifer practiced self-validation during a difficult interaction with her mother, who had made critical comments about Jennifer's life choices. Jennifer's automatic response was to feel angry and then immediately criticize herself for being "too sensitive" and "overreacting" to her mother's input.

Using self-validation, Jennifer instead acknowledged: "I'm feeling angry and hurt by my mother's comments. This makes sense because I value her approval and these comments feel critical of choices that are important to me. It's natural to feel upset when someone I care about expresses disapproval of my life. I can be kind to myself while feeling these difficult emotions."

Validating others without losing yourself

Individuals with quiet BPD often struggle with validation boundaries—they may provide excessive validation that enables others' problematic behaviors, or they may invalidate others' experiences because they're afraid of being emotionally overwhelmed. Learning to validate appropriately means offering understanding without automatically adopting others' emotional experiences or taking responsibility for fixing their problems.

Healthy validation includes:

- Acknowledging the other person's emotional experience
- Expressing understanding of why they might feel that way
- Offering support without taking responsibility for their feelings

- Maintaining your own emotional boundaries during the interaction

Case example: Validating without enabling

When Tom's friend called to complain about work difficulties for the third time that week, Tom's traditional response was to spend hours listening, offering solutions, and taking on his friend's emotional distress as if it were his own responsibility. This pattern left Tom emotionally drained while not actually helping his friend develop better coping skills.

Using appropriate validation boundaries, Tom responded: "It sounds like work has been really stressful for you lately, and I can understand why you'd feel frustrated with these ongoing problems. What kind of support would be most helpful for you right now?" This response acknowledged his friend's experience while maintaining appropriate boundaries about Tom's role in addressing the problems.

The SET method for difficult conversations

The SET method—Support, Empathy, Truth—provides a framework for having difficult conversations while maintaining both connection and authenticity. This approach was originally developed for communicating with individuals with BPD, but it works effectively for anyone learning to balance emotional support with honest communication.

Support: Begin difficult conversations by acknowledging your care for the relationship and your desire to work through challenges together. This creates emotional safety that allows the other person to hear difficult feedback without feeling attacked or rejected.

Empathy: Express understanding of the other person's perspective or emotional experience, even if you disagree with their behavior or decisions. This validation helps prevent defensive responses and creates space for productive dialogue.

Truth: Share your authentic thoughts, feelings, or needs clearly and directly, without minimizing or apologizing for your perspective. This is where individuals with quiet BPD often struggle—they may excel at providing support and empathy but struggle to share their truth directly.

Case example: Family boundary setting

Lisa's relationship with her sister had become increasingly strained due to her sister's pattern of calling during emotional crises and expecting Lisa to drop everything to provide support. Lisa had been providing this support for years while building internal resentment about the one-sided nature of their relationship.

Using the SET method, Lisa addressed the pattern:

Support: "I care about you and want to continue being someone you can turn to when you're struggling."

Empathy: "I understand that you're going through a difficult time with work and relationships, and I can see why you'd want to talk through these challenges."

Truth: "I need us to find a way for me to support you that doesn't require me to be available immediately whenever you call. I'd like to set up regular times when we can talk, and I need you to check if I'm available before launching into crisis conversations."

Lisa's sister initially responded defensively, but the support and empathy components of Lisa's message helped her hear the truth without feeling completely rejected. Over time, they developed a more balanced relationship that honored both of their needs.

Boundary setting for people-pleasers

Boundary setting represents one of the most challenging skills for individuals with quiet BPD because it requires risking disapproval and potential relationship conflict. However, appropriate boundaries are essential for authentic relationships—they allow others to know your genuine limits and preferences rather than interacting with your people-pleasing persona.

Understanding boundary confusion

Many individuals with quiet BPD struggle to distinguish between healthy boundaries and selfish demands. Their childhood experiences often taught them that their needs were secondary to others' comfort, creating confusion about when it's appropriate to prioritize their own well-being.

Healthy boundaries:

- Communicate your limits clearly and kindly
- Protect your physical and emotional well-being
- Allow others to make informed decisions about how to interact with you
- Support authentic relationships by preventing resentment and emotional exhaustion

Boundary violations disguised as niceness:

- Saying yes when you mean no to avoid disappointing others
- Taking responsibility for others' emotional reactions to your boundaries
- Automatically prioritizing others' needs over your own well-being
- Avoiding boundaries because you're afraid others won't like you

The gradual boundary development process

Setting boundaries feels terrifying for quiet BPD individuals because they fear that others will leave if they stop being perfectly accommodating. The most effective approach involves gradually increasing boundary firmness while building evidence that relationships can survive and even improve when you express your genuine limits.

Step 1: Internal boundary recognition Before you can communicate boundaries to others, you need to identify what your actual limits are. This requires paying attention to situations that create resentment, exhaustion, or internal conflict.

Step 2: Small boundary practice Begin with low-stakes boundary setting that feels manageable. This might involve declining minor social invitations when you need rest, or expressing preferences about restaurants or activities.

Step 3: Emotional preparation Expect that boundary setting will trigger anxiety about rejection and disapproval. Prepare self-soothing strategies and supportive relationships to help you tolerate these difficult emotions.

Step 4: Clear, kind communication Express boundaries directly using "I" statements that focus on your needs rather than criticizing others' requests. "I need to leave by 9 PM" rather than "You always keep me too late."

Step 5: Boundary maintenance The most difficult part of boundary setting involves maintaining your limits when others push back or express disappointment. This requires tolerating others' emotional reactions without automatically changing your boundaries to make them more comfortable.

Assertiveness training for conflict-avoidant personalities

Traditional assertiveness training assumes that individuals want to express their needs but lack the skills to do so effectively. Quiet BPD individuals often possess excellent assertiveness skills intellectually but struggle to use them because they're terrified of the conflict or rejection that assertiveness might create.

Reframing assertiveness for anxiety-sensitive individuals

111

Dr. Patricia Williams explains that assertiveness for quiet BPD individuals requires addressing the underlying anxiety about interpersonal consequences rather than simply teaching communication techniques: "These individuals often know how to be assertive—they can role-play assertive responses perfectly in therapy. The challenge is tolerating the emotional vulnerability that real assertiveness requires."

Assertiveness as relationship building

For conflict-avoidant individuals, it helps to reframe assertiveness as a relationship-building skill rather than a conflict-creating one. When you express your authentic needs and preferences, you're giving others the information they need to have genuine relationships with you rather than relationships with your people-pleasing persona.

Case example: Assertiveness in friendship

Karen had maintained a friendship for five years by consistently adapting to her friend's preferences for activities, conversation topics, and social schedules. While this strategy prevented conflict, it also prevented Karen from discovering whether her friend could enjoy activities that Karen preferred or appreciate conversations about topics that interested her.

Karen's first assertiveness experiment involved suggesting a hiking trip instead of their usual shopping excursions. She prepared for potential rejection by reminding herself that if her friend couldn't accommodate any of Karen's preferences, the friendship was based on Karen's performance rather than genuine connection.

Her friend's enthusiastic response surprised Karen—she had been interested in hiking but had assumed Karen preferred shopping because that's what they always did. This experience taught Karen that her people-pleasing strategy had been preventing mutual discovery rather than protecting the relationship.

Family workshop exercises for healing relationships

Many individuals with quiet BPD come from family systems that inadvertently reinforced emotional suppression and people-pleasing patterns. Healing these relationships often requires family-wide changes in communication patterns rather than individual changes alone.

Family communication assessment

The first step in family healing involves honest assessment of current communication patterns:

- How does your family handle disagreement and conflict?
- Who takes responsibility for managing everyone else's emotions?
- What topics are considered off-limits or too sensitive to discuss?
- How does your family respond when members express strong emotions?
- What are the unspoken rules about emotional expression in your family?

Gradual family system changes

Family communication patterns developed over years or decades and require patience and persistence to change. The most effective approach involves introducing small changes gradually rather than attempting to transform all family interactions immediately.

Exercise 1: Emotion check-ins During family gatherings, practice brief emotion check-ins where each family member shares how they're currently feeling without trying to fix or change each other's emotional states. This normalizes emotional expression and gives family members practice with authentic sharing.

Exercise 2: Appreciation and concern sharing Set aside time during family interactions for each person to share one thing they appreciate about another family member and one concern or request they have.

This creates structured opportunities for both positive expression and gentle feedback.

Exercise 3: Conflict resolution practice When disagreements arise, practice using the SET method as a family communication tool. Each person takes turns expressing support for the relationship, empathy for others' perspectives, and their own truth about the situation.

Case example: Family transformation

The Johnson family had maintained harmony for twenty years through elaborate conflict avoidance and emotional suppression. Everyone was polite, considerate, and careful not to upset anyone else. However, when their daughter Sarah began therapy for quiet BPD, she realized that their family's "closeness" was actually preventing genuine intimacy.

Sarah initiated family conversations about their communication patterns, expressing her desire for more authentic relationships with her parents and siblings. Initially, her family members were uncomfortable with her requests for more emotional honesty, fearing that direct communication would damage their relationships.

Over several months, they gradually practiced new communication patterns. Sarah's father shared his anxiety about work pressures instead of pretending everything was fine. Her mother expressed her feelings about being the family's emotional caretaker. Sarah's brother talked about feeling pressure to be perfect rather than maintaining his achievement-focused persona.

These conversations were often difficult and emotionally intense, but they led to deeper family connections and reduced the emotional burden that each family member had been carrying individually. The family learned that relationships could become stronger through authentic expression rather than protective performance.

Practical communication tools

Building authentic communication skills requires practice and specific techniques for managing the anxiety that vulnerability creates. The following tools provide concrete strategies for moving from withdrawal to expression:

The pause technique: When you notice yourself automatically editing your responses, take a brief pause to check in with your authentic thoughts and feelings before responding. This creates space for conscious choice rather than automatic people-pleasing.

The graduated honesty approach: Begin with low-stakes honesty practice and gradually work toward more vulnerable sharing. Start by expressing genuine preferences about minor topics before progressing to sharing important emotions or concerns.

The relationship inventory: Regularly assess your relationships for authenticity. Are there relationships where you feel safe being genuine? Are there patterns where you consistently edit yourself? Use this information to guide your communication practice.

The emotional courage building: Develop tolerance for the anxiety that authentic expression creates. Practice self-soothing techniques, seek support from understanding friends, and remind yourself that temporary discomfort is worthwhile for authentic relationships.

Moving beyond silence

The journey from silence to expression requires tremendous courage because it means risking the rejection and abandonment that emotional suppression was designed to prevent. However, the relationships that survive this transition become infinitely more satisfying and sustainable than those built on people-pleasing and emotional performance.

Learning to speak your truth doesn't mean expressing every thought and feeling without consideration for others. It means developing the capacity to be authentic within appropriate boundaries, to express your genuine self while remaining caring and considerate toward others.

This balance—authenticity with kindness—represents the goal of healthy communication for individuals recovering from quiet BPD.

Core lessons learned

- Authentic communication requires reconnecting with genuine thoughts and feelings before attempting to share them with others
- Self-validation provides the internal foundation needed for expressing authentic emotions without depending entirely on others' responses
- The SET method (Support, Empathy, Truth) provides a framework for difficult conversations that maintains both connection and honesty
- Boundary setting protects authentic relationships by preventing resentment and emotional exhaustion that come from constant people-pleasing
- Assertiveness for quiet BPD individuals requires addressing anxiety about interpersonal consequences rather than simply teaching communication techniques
- Family healing often requires system-wide changes in communication patterns rather than individual changes alone
- Building communication skills requires graduated practice and tolerance for the anxiety that vulnerability initially creates

Chapter 12: Rewiring the inner critic

The voice started at 5:47 AM, the moment Sarah's alarm went off. "You should have gone to bed earlier. Now you'll be tired all day and everyone will notice you're not functioning properly. You're so undisciplined." By the time she reached for her toothbrush, the voice had catalogued seventeen ways she'd already failed before 6 AM. The voice wasn't external—no one else could hear it. But it was relentless, merciless, and had been Sarah's primary internal companion for twenty-eight years.

This inner critic—that harsh, demanding voice that judges every thought, feeling, and action—represents one of the most destructive aspects of quiet BPD. Unlike the dramatic external conflicts that characterize classic BPD presentations, quiet BPD individuals wage daily battles against an internal enemy that knows exactly which buttons to push and never takes a break from criticism. Learning to rewire this critic isn't about positive thinking or self-affirmations (though those can help)—it's about understanding why this voice developed and systematically replacing its destructive messages with more balanced, realistic assessments.

The shame spiral and self-punishment cycle

The inner critic in quiet BPD operates through what clinicians call "shame spirals"—cascading cycles of self-criticism that gain momentum and intensity until they feel inescapable. These spirals often begin with minor triggers—a colleague's neutral expression, a friend's delayed text response, or a small mistake at work—but quickly escalate into comprehensive character assassinations.

Consider Maria, a 32-year-old graphic designer whose shame spiral began when she noticed a typo in an email she'd sent to her team. Within minutes, her inner critic had constructed an elaborate narrative: "You can't even proofread a simple email. Everyone will think you're careless and unprofessional. You don't deserve this job. You're a fraud and eventually everyone will figure it out. You should just quit before they fire you."

The shame spiral follows a predictable pattern:

1. **Triggering event** - Something happens that activates sensitivity to rejection or criticism
2. **Initial self-criticism** - The inner critic identifies the "mistake" or "flaw"
3. **Catastrophic thinking** - The criticism expands to predict dire consequences
4. **Character assassination** - The focus shifts from behavior to identity ("I'm a failure")
5. **Evidence gathering** - The mind searches for additional proof of inadequacy
6. **Future forecasting** - Predictions about how this flaw will ruin future opportunities
7. **Self-punishment** - Emotional or behavioral consequences for being "defective"

The self-punishment aspect of this cycle is particularly destructive for quiet BPD individuals. Unlike classic BPD presentations where self-punishment might involve obvious self-harm or dramatic gestures, quiet BPD self-punishment is often invisible to others:

*   **Emotional self-harm** - Deliberately dwelling on painful thoughts or memories
*   **Social withdrawal** - Isolating yourself as punishment for perceived failures
*   **Opportunity sabotage** - Avoiding positive experiences because you don't "deserve" them
*   **Perfectionist punishment** - Setting impossibly high standards then criticizing yourself for falling short
*   **Relationship testing** - Pushing others away to confirm your belief that you're unlovable

Understanding the critic's development

The harsh inner critic doesn't develop randomly—it's usually an internalized version of critical voices from childhood, combined with the brain's attempt to prevent future rejection or abandonment. For quiet BPD individuals, this critic often developed as a survival mechanism in environments where emotional expression or authentic selfhood felt dangerous.

Take David's experience growing up in a high-achieving family where his parents, both physicians, emphasized academic excellence and emotional restraint. Any display of strong emotions was met with subtle but clear disapproval—sighs, eye rolls, or comments about being "dramatic" or "too sensitive." David learned that his emotional intensity was problematic and developed an internal voice that constantly monitored and criticized his emotional responses.

By adulthood, David's inner critic had become more sophisticated and harsh than his parents' original criticism. It had learned exactly which self-attacks would be most effective: "You're too needy. No one wants to deal with your emotions. You're exhausting to be around. Just keep it to yourself." This voice felt protective—it was trying to prevent the rejection and criticism that David had experienced as a child. But it had become so powerful that it was now creating the isolation it was designed to prevent.

The critic's messages often contain three core themes that reflect childhood emotional wounds:

Defectiveness - "Something is fundamentally wrong with you"
Unlovability - "You're too much for people to handle" **Inadequacy** - "You'll never be good enough"

These themes aren't random—they directly reflect the types of invalidation that many quiet BPD individuals experienced during their formative years. The critic isn't being mean for no reason; it's trying to protect you from experiencing those painful childhood feelings again. Unfortunately, its protection strategy involves constant vigilance and preemptive self-attack, which creates the very pain it's trying to prevent.

Cognitive restructuring for the perfectionist mind

Traditional cognitive restructuring teaches people to identify negative thoughts and replace them with more balanced alternatives. For quiet BPD individuals, this approach requires modifications because their perfectionist minds often resist anything that seems like "lowering standards" or "making excuses." The key is learning to distinguish between **helpful evaluation** (which improves performance) and **destructive criticism** (which paralyzes and demoralizes).

The perfectionist's dilemma

Jennifer, a 29-year-old attorney, struggled with cognitive restructuring because she feared that being less critical of herself would make her lazy or careless. "If I don't push myself hard, I'll become mediocre," she explained. "My standards are what make me successful." This belief system is common among high-functioning quiet BPD individuals—they credit their harsh self-criticism with their achievements and fear that self-compassion will lead to decline.

The solution involves distinguishing between **productive self-evaluation** and **destructive self-attack**:

Productive evaluation:

- Focuses on specific behaviors rather than global character flaws
- Identifies concrete steps for improvement
- Maintains perspective about the significance of mistakes
- Includes recognition of successes alongside areas for growth
- Motivates rather than paralyzes

Destructive self-attack:

- Makes sweeping generalizations about your worth as a person
- Focuses on punishment rather than problem-solving
- Catastrophizes the consequences of minor mistakes
- Ignores successes and focuses exclusively on flaws

- Creates shame and paralysis rather than motivation

Jennifer learned to catch her inner critic in action and ask: "Is this evaluation helping me improve, or is it just making me feel terrible?" When she noticed self-attacks, she would consciously redirect to productive evaluation: Instead of "I'm such an idiot for missing that deadline," she would think, "I missed this deadline because I underestimated the time needed. Next time I'll build in a buffer and check my timeline midway through the project."

The thought record technique for quiet BPD

The traditional thought record—a cognitive behavioral therapy tool for examining thoughts and emotions—requires adaptation for quiet BPD because these individuals often have difficulty accessing their automatic thoughts. Their thoughts move so quickly from trigger to self-attack that they don't notice the intermediate steps.

Modified thought record process:

1. **Situation identification** - What was happening when you started feeling bad?
2. **Emotion tracking** - What emotions are you experiencing and how intense are they?
3. **Body scan** - Where do you feel these emotions physically?
4. **Slow-motion replay** - Go back through the situation slowly to catch the rapid-fire thoughts
5. **Critic voice identification** - What is your inner critic saying about this situation?
6. **Evidence examination** - What evidence supports and contradicts this criticism?
7. **Balanced perspective** - What would you tell a good friend in this situation?
8. **Action planning** - What concrete steps can you take to address any real issues?

Lisa used this modified process after a difficult interaction with her supervisor. Initially, she could only identify feeling "terrible" and

121

thinking "I'm incompetent." Using the slow-motion replay, she discovered a rapid sequence of self-attacks: "She looked annoyed. I must have said something wrong. I always say the wrong thing. I don't belong in this job. Everyone thinks I'm stupid."

The evidence examination revealed that her supervisor had seemed distracted throughout their entire conversation, not just during Lisa's contributions. Lisa also remembered receiving positive feedback from this same supervisor just the week before. The balanced perspective question helped her consider: "If my friend told me her boss seemed distracted during one conversation, would I conclude that my friend was incompetent?" Obviously not.

Self-compassion practices that work for skeptics

Many quiet BPD individuals resist self-compassion practices because they seem "weak," "self-indulgent," or potentially harmful to performance. The key is presenting self-compassion not as lowering standards, but as providing the emotional safety needed for optimal functioning and learning.

Self-compassion for high achievers

Research shows that self-compassion actually improves performance by reducing the anxiety and shame that interfere with learning and risk-taking. Athletes who practice self-compassion bounce back more quickly from mistakes. Students who treat themselves kindly show greater motivation to study after poor test performance. Workers who forgive themselves for errors are less likely to repeat them.

Dr. Lisa Chen worked with Marcus, a 35-year-old financial analyst, who initially refused self-compassion practices because he believed they would make him "soft" and reduce his competitive edge. She reframed self-compassion as "performance optimization": "You wouldn't yell at and berate a teammate who made a mistake, because that would hurt team performance. You're currently doing to yourself what you would never do to someone else on your team."

The three components of self-compassion adapted for quiet BPD:

Self-kindness - Treating yourself with the same gentleness you'd show a good friend experiencing difficulty. For quiet BPD individuals, this often means simply stopping active self-attack rather than immediately jumping to positive self-talk.

Common humanity - Recognizing that struggle, mistakes, and imperfection are part of the human experience rather than personal failures. This counters the isolation that comes from believing you're uniquely flawed or inadequate.

Mindful awareness - Observing difficult emotions without immediately trying to fix, change, or judge them. For over-controlling quiet BPD individuals, this means practicing allowing difficult feelings to exist without instantly mobilizing problem-solving or self-improvement efforts.

Practical self-compassion exercises:

The best friend technique - When you notice harsh self-criticism, ask "What would I say to my best friend if they were in this exact situation?" Then try to offer yourself the same support.

The compassionate body posture - Place your hand on your heart, take a few deep breaths, and remind yourself "This is a moment of difficulty. Difficulty is part of life. May I be kind to myself during this hard time."

The self-compassion break - During difficult moments, pause and acknowledge: "This hurts. I'm not the only person who has experienced this. I can be gentle with myself right now."

The compassionate reframe - Transform self-attacks into compassionate observations: Instead of "I'm so stupid," try "I'm having a hard time with this, and that's understandable given the complexity of the situation."

Values clarification for authentic living

Many quiet BPD individuals have spent so much energy trying to be what others want that they've lost touch with their authentic values and priorities. They can articulate what they "should" care about or what seems socially appropriate, but struggle to identify what actually matters to them personally.

The values confusion problem

Rachel, a 31-year-old social worker, could easily list values that seemed appropriate for her profession: helping others, social justice, compassion. But when pressed to identify what she personally found most meaningful, she became confused and anxious. "I don't know what I actually value," she admitted. "I've spent so long figuring out what other people want from me that I don't know what I want for myself."

This values confusion is common in quiet BPD because the condition often develops in families or environments where individual preferences were discouraged or ignored in favor of family harmony or social expectations. Children learn to suppress their authentic interests and adopt values that earn approval, eventually losing touch with their genuine preferences.

Values clarification exercises:

The time machine exercise - If you could go back to age seven and spend the day doing anything you wanted, what would you choose? This helps bypass adult "shoulds" and reconnect with authentic interests.

The deathbed test - When you're very old, looking back on your life, what would you want to be able to say about how you lived? This cuts through social expectations to identify what you actually find meaningful.

The energy audit - Track which activities energize you versus which drain you over the course of a week. Often, activities aligned with authentic values feel energizing even when they're challenging.

The jealousy investigation - What kinds of lives or achievements trigger envy in you? Jealousy often points toward values you haven't acknowledged or pursued.

The childhood dream review - What did you want to be when you grew up, and what values were embedded in those dreams? A child who wanted to be a teacher might value learning, growth, or helping others develop.

Identity work beyond the false self

Quiet BPD often involves developing what psychologists call a "false self"—a carefully constructed persona designed to earn approval and avoid rejection. This false self might be highly successful and socially skilled, but it feels hollow because it's not connected to authentic desires, emotions, or experiences.

Understanding the false self construction

The false self develops as protection against environments where authentic self-expression feels dangerous. Kevin, a 28-year-old marketing manager, described his false self as "a really good actor playing the role of a successful, happy person." He had become so skilled at this performance that even close friends saw him as naturally confident and easygoing, while internally he felt anxious, empty, and disconnected from his supposed life.

The false self often includes:

- **Personality traits** you've developed because they seem socially valuable
- **Interests and hobbies** you've adopted to fit in with certain groups

- **Career choices** made to impress others rather than satisfy personal interests
- **Relationship patterns** designed to maintain others' approval rather than express authentic needs
- **Emotional expressions** that match what seems appropriate rather than what you actually feel

The authentic self recovery process

Reconnecting with authentic identity requires patience because the false self often developed over many years and may have become so automatic that it feels "natural." The process involves:

Authentic experience tracking - Notice moments when you feel most "like yourself"—when you're not performing or adapting to others' expectations. What are you doing? Who are you with? What aspects of yourself are you expressing?

False self recognition - Begin identifying moments when you're "acting" rather than being authentic. This isn't about judging the performance, but about developing awareness of when you're adapting versus expressing.

Gradual authenticity experiments - Start expressing small aspects of your authentic self in low-risk situations. Share a genuine opinion, express a real emotion, or pursue an activity that interests you personally rather than socially.

Identity integration - Work toward integrating authentic aspects of yourself with the social skills and achievements of your false self. The goal isn't to destroy everything you've built, but to make it more genuinely representative of who you are.

Daily practices for emotional stability

Rewiring the inner critic and developing authentic identity requires consistent daily practices rather than occasional therapeutic insights. The practices that work best for quiet BPD individuals are those that can be integrated into existing routines without feeling overwhelming or time-consuming.

Morning emotional check-in routine

Instead of immediately jumping into productivity or problem-solving, spend five minutes each morning checking in with your actual emotional state:

1. **Body scan** - Notice physical sensations without trying to change them
2. **Emotion identification** - Name what you're feeling without judging it as good or bad
3. **Need assessment** - Ask what you need today to feel emotionally stable
4. **Intention setting** - Choose one way you'll be kind to yourself during the day
5. **Critic monitoring** - Notice if your inner critic is particularly active and remind yourself that thoughts aren't facts

Evening self-compassion practice

Before bed, spend a few minutes reviewing the day with kindness:

1. **Achievement acknowledgment** - Identify at least three things you accomplished, no matter how small
2. **Difficulty recognition** - Acknowledge any challenges you faced without immediately trying to solve them
3. **Self-forgiveness** - If you made mistakes, practice offering yourself the same forgiveness you'd give a good friend
4. **Gratitude for effort** - Appreciate the effort you put into your day, regardless of outcomes
5. **Tomorrow's intention** - Set a gentle intention for how you want to treat yourself tomorrow

Midday reality checks

Set a daily reminder to pause and check in with your inner dialogue:

- Is your inner critic being particularly harsh today?
- Are you treating yourself the way you'd treat someone you care about?
- What would change if you spoke to yourself more kindly?
- What do you need right now to feel more balanced?

These practices work because they interrupt the automatic patterns of self-criticism and create space for more balanced self-assessment. They're not about forced positivity or pretending everything is fine—they're about developing a more realistic and compassionate relationship with yourself.

The goal of rewiring the inner critic isn't to eliminate self-evaluation or lower your standards. It's to develop an internal voice that motivates rather than demoralizes, that recognizes both strengths and areas for growth, and that treats you as a human being deserving of kindness rather than as an enemy to be defeated.

Changing deeply ingrained patterns of self-criticism requires both patience and persistence. The inner critic developed over many years as protection against rejection and criticism, so it won't disappear overnight. But with consistent practice, you can develop a more balanced internal voice—one that maintains high standards while also providing the emotional safety needed for growth, learning, and authentic relationships.

You'll know you're making progress when you notice the critic's voice becoming less frequent and less harsh, when you can catch and redirect self-attacks before they spiral out of control, and when you begin treating yourself with some of the same kindness you naturally offer to others you care about.

- The inner critic in quiet BPD operates through shame spirals that escalate from minor triggers to comprehensive self-attacks
- This harsh internal voice developed as protection against childhood invalidation but now creates the pain it was designed to prevent

- Cognitive restructuring for perfectionists requires distinguishing between productive evaluation and destructive self-attack
- Self-compassion improves rather than hinders performance by reducing anxiety and shame that interfere with learning
- Values clarification helps reconnect with authentic interests that may have been suppressed in favor of social approval
- Identity work involves recognizing the false self while gradually expressing more authentic aspects of personality
- Daily practices for emotional stability include morning check-ins, evening self-compassion, and midday reality checks that interrupt automatic self-criticism patterns

Chapter 13: Relationships that heal

The dating app notification chimed at 3:47 PM on a Tuesday, and Sarah's stomach immediately clenched. Another match. Another opportunity for connection that felt simultaneously thrilling and terrifying. She had been single for eight months—the longest stretch since high school—not because she didn't want a relationship, but because dating with quiet BPD felt like navigating a minefield blindfolded. How do you get close to someone when you're not sure who you actually are underneath all the people-pleasing? How do you build intimacy when your deepest fear is that someone will discover you're "too much" and leave?

Relationships represent both the greatest challenge and the most powerful healing opportunity for individuals with quiet BPD. The same emotional intensity and sensitivity that make relationships feel dangerous also create the capacity for extraordinary depth, empathy, and connection. Learning to build relationships that heal rather than trigger requires understanding your patterns, developing new skills, and gradually taking the emotional risks that authentic intimacy demands.

Dating with quiet BPD

The dating process presents unique challenges for individuals with quiet BPD because it involves presenting yourself authentically to strangers while managing the intense emotions that potential rejection can trigger. Traditional dating advice assumes people know who they are and what they want—assumptions that don't always hold true for someone still discovering their authentic self.

The timing question

Maria had been in therapy for eighteen months, working on her tendency toward people-pleasing and emotional suppression, when she began considering dating again. Her therapist posed a challenging question: "Can you be alone with yourself comfortably for at least a few hours without feeling panicked or empty?" Maria realized she couldn't. She still needed constant external validation and stimulation to feel stable, which meant she wasn't ready to enter relationships from a place of choice rather than desperation.

The timing of dating during quiet BPD recovery involves several considerations:

- **Identity stability** - Do you have some sense of your authentic preferences, values, and interests, or are you still primarily defined by what others want from you?
- **Emotional regulation** - Can you manage disappointment, anxiety, and excitement without completely falling apart or shutting down?
- **Independence capacity** - Can you enjoy your own company and manage daily life without requiring constant relationship input?
- **Boundary awareness** - Do you know what your limits are and can you communicate them, or do you automatically defer to others' preferences?

This doesn't mean you need to be "perfect" before dating—no one is ever completely healed or self-aware. But having some foundation of self-knowledge and emotional regulation skills makes it more likely that relationships will add to your life rather than become your primary source of stability.

The disclosure dilemma

One of the most anxiety-provoking aspects of dating with quiet BPD involves deciding what to share about your mental health and when. Unlike more visible conditions, quiet BPD can remain hidden for months or even years in relationships, but this secrecy often creates additional stress and authenticity barriers.

Jason struggled with this decision throughout his six-month relationship with Emma. He desperately wanted to explain why he sometimes seemed distant after social events (emotional exhaustion from masking), why he occasionally needed excessive reassurance about their relationship (abandonment fears), and why he had such strong reactions to criticism (rejection sensitivity). But he feared that disclosing his quiet BPD diagnosis would scare Emma away or change how she saw him.

Guidelines for disclosure decisions:

Early dating (first few months): Focus on sharing your authentic self rather than diagnostic labels. Mention that you're sensitive, need some alone time to recharge, or are working on communication skills in therapy. This gives potential partners accurate information without overwhelming them with medical terminology.

Developing relationships (3-6 months): If the relationship is progressing toward seriousness, consider sharing more specific information about your patterns and needs. Explain your tendency toward people-pleasing, your sensitivity to criticism, or your need for reassurance during difficult times.

Committed relationships (6+ months): In serious relationships, sharing your quiet BPD diagnosis can actually strengthen intimacy by helping your partner understand your experiences and needs. Frame it as information that helps them support you rather than a problem they need to fix.

The authentic dating approach

Traditional dating advice often encourages people to "put their best foot forward," but this approach can be problematic for quiet BPD individuals who already struggle with authenticity. The goal is finding someone who appreciates your genuine self rather than someone who likes your performance.

Rachel experimented with radical honesty in her online dating profile: "I'm an introvert who needs downtime after social events, I'm working on speaking up for what I need in relationships, and I tend to be highly sensitive to others' emotions. I'm looking for someone who appreciates depth and isn't afraid of real conversations." She received fewer matches than with her previous "bubbly and easy-going" persona, but the conversations were dramatically more meaningful.

Practical dating strategies:

- **Choose activities that reflect your authentic interests** rather than what seems most socially acceptable
- **Practice expressing genuine opinions** about movies, restaurants, politics, or other topics instead of agreeing with everything your date says
- **Share appropriate vulnerabilities** gradually rather than maintaining perfect composure throughout the relationship development
- **Pay attention to how you feel** around different people rather than focusing solely on how much they seem to like you
- **Notice red flags** like partners who discourage your therapy, criticize your sensitivity, or pressure you to be different than you are

Parenting when you're healing

For individuals with quiet BPD who become parents, the challenges multiply exponentially. Parenting triggers every abandonment fear, perfectionist tendency, and emotional regulation difficulty while simultaneously requiring you to model healthy emotional expression for your children. The good news is that working on your quiet BPD recovery can actually make you a more attuned, emotionally available parent than you might have been otherwise.

Breaking intergenerational patterns

Lisa recognized the patterns from her own childhood playing out with her five-year-old daughter: the subtle discouragement of strong emotions, the emphasis on being "good" and "easy," and the unspoken message that love was conditional on appropriate behavior. She was recreating the same emotional environment that had contributed to her own quiet BPD development, despite her conscious intention to be different.

The key to breaking these patterns involves conscious attention to your automatic responses to your children's emotional expressions:

Traditional responses that reinforce emotional suppression:

- "You're fine, it's not that bad"
- "Big boys/girls don't cry"
- "You're being too dramatic"
- "Calm down and then we'll talk"
- "I like you better when you're happy"

Responses that validate emotions while teaching regulation:

- "You're really upset about this. That makes sense."
- "It's okay to feel angry. Let's figure out what to do with this feeling."
- "You seem overwhelmed. What would help you feel better?"
- "I can see this is hard for you. I'm here to help."
- "All feelings are okay. Some behaviors need limits."

Modeling emotional authenticity

Children learn emotional regulation more from what they observe than from what they're told. Lisa began practicing appropriate emotional authenticity with her daughter—sharing when she felt sad, expressing excitement about things she genuinely enjoyed, and admitting when she made mistakes.

"Mommy made a mistake when I got frustrated about the messy kitchen," Lisa would say. "I raised my voice, and that probably felt scary. I was stressed about other things, but that's not your fault. I'm going to take some deep breaths and try again."

This modeling taught her daughter that emotions are normal, mistakes are fixable, and adults can take responsibility for their behavior while still being loving and trustworthy.

Self-care as parenting strategy

Parents with quiet BPD often feel guilty about taking time for self-care, believing that good parents should be completely focused on their children's needs. In reality, modeling self-care teaches children that their own needs matter and that taking care of yourself allows you to better care for others.

Lisa established several non-negotiable self-care practices:

- Twenty minutes of alone time each day after her daughter went to bed
- Weekly therapy appointments that she never cancelled for non-emergencies
- Monthly solo activities that brought her joy
- Daily check-ins with her own emotional state before responding to her daughter's needs

Her daughter learned that adults have needs too, that it's normal to take breaks when you're overwhelmed, and that self-care is a life skill rather than selfishness.

Building friendship networks that understand

Many individuals with quiet BPD struggle with friendships because they exhaust themselves maintaining relationships through people-pleasing while rarely receiving the emotional support they actually need. Building friendships that sustain rather than drain requires learning to show up authentically and seek out people who can handle your genuine self.

The friendship energy audit

Marcus realized that most of his friendships left him feeling drained rather than energized. He was always the listener, the helper, the one who remembered everyone's problems and provided support during crises. His friends saw him as stable and reliable, but he rarely felt comfortable sharing his own struggles or asking for support.

The friendship audit involves honestly assessing your current relationships:

Energy-giving friendships:

- You can be authentic about both positive and negative experiences
- Conversations feel balanced—both people share and both people listen
- You feel accepted for who you are rather than what you provide
- Conflicts can be addressed directly without threatening the relationship
- You feel energized or neutral after spending time together

Energy-draining friendships:

- You feel like you're performing or managing the other person's emotions
- Conversations focus primarily on their problems with little reciprocal interest in yours
- You feel judged or criticized for your sensitivity or needs
- Conflicts get avoided or result in you automatically apologizing and accommodating
- You feel exhausted or depleted after interactions

This doesn't mean immediately ending all challenging relationships, but it does mean becoming more intentional about where you invest your social energy and gradually cultivating relationships that feel more reciprocal.

Finding your people

Individuals with quiet BPD often connect well with others who have some experience with mental health challenges, therapy, or personal growth work. These people tend to be more comfortable with emotional depth and less likely to judge sensitivity or struggles.

Places to meet emotionally mature people:

- Therapy or support groups (with appropriate boundaries about dual relationships)
- Volunteer organizations focused on causes you care about
- Classes or workshops related to personal growth, mindfulness, or creative expression
- Online communities focused on mental health, highly sensitive people, or specific interests
- Activities that attract introspective or emotionally aware individuals

The key is showing up as your authentic self from the beginning rather than waiting until you're "comfortable enough" to be genuine. This filters out people who can't handle your real personality while attracting those who appreciate depth and authenticity.

Case example: Friendship transformation

Jennifer had maintained the same group of college friends for ten years, but realized that she had never shared her struggles with anxiety, her therapy experiences, or her actual opinions about many topics they discussed. She was friendly with everyone but truly known by no one.

She began an experiment: over the course of six months, she gradually shared more authentic aspects of herself with each friend. With some friends, this created deeper connections as they reciprocated with their own vulnerabilities. With others, the relationships naturally faded as it became clear they preferred her supportive persona to her complete self.

The process was initially painful—Jennifer grieved the loss of some relationships and felt anxious about the increased vulnerability. But the friendships that survived became dramatically more satisfying and supportive. She discovered that several of her friends had been struggling with similar issues but hadn't felt safe sharing them either.

Support network development

Building a support network involves more than just having friends—it requires cultivating relationships with different people who can meet different needs and provide various types of support during difficult times.

Types of support needed:

Emotional support - People who can listen without trying to fix, validate your experiences, and provide comfort during difficult times

Practical support - People who can help with concrete needs like transportation, childcare, or household tasks during crises

Informational support - People who have knowledge or experience relevant to your challenges and can provide guidance or resources

Social support - People who include you in activities and help prevent isolation

Professional support - Therapists, doctors, and other professionals who provide clinical care

Most people need different individuals filling these roles rather than expecting any single relationship to meet all support needs. Your romantic partner might provide emotional support but not practical help. A friend might be great for social connection but not the right person for deep emotional conversations.

Creating a support map

Draw a circle with yourself in the center and add rings moving outward. Place the people in your life in different rings based on how much support they currently provide:

- **Inner circle** - People you can call at 3 AM during a crisis
- **Middle circle** - People you see regularly and can share moderate vulnerabilities with
- **Outer circle** - Acquaintances and casual friends who provide social connection

Most people discover that their inner circle is smaller than they'd like and their outer circle larger than necessary. Building a stronger support network involves gradually deepening some middle circle relationships and being more selective about energy investment in outer circle connections.

Case example: Support network building

After her divorce, Rebecca realized that most of her social connections had been through her ex-husband and that she had no one to call during her frequent anxiety attacks. She systematically worked on building different types of support:

- **Emotional support**: She joined a therapy group and developed closer relationships with two women who understood anxiety and depression
- **Practical support**: She connected with neighbors who could help with childcare emergencies and found a reliable handyman for household issues
- **Informational support**: She found online communities for single mothers and individuals with anxiety disorders
- **Social support**: She joined a hiking group and book club to prevent isolation
- **Professional support**: She established relationships with a therapist, psychiatrist, and primary care doctor

This network development took nearly two years, but it provided Rebecca with multiple sources of support that prevented her from becoming too dependent on any single relationship while ensuring her needs could be met during difficult periods.

Couple's exercises for partners navigating quiet BPD

When one partner has quiet BPD, both people need education and tools for building healthy relationship patterns. The challenges often involve helping the quiet BPD partner express their authentic needs while helping the other partner understand the hidden emotional intensity they're dealing with.

The emotional temperature check

Many couples dealing with quiet BPD develop communication patterns where the non-BPD partner remains unaware of their partner's emotional states until problems reach crisis levels. The emotional temperature check creates regular opportunities for authentic communication about internal experiences.

Daily check-in process:

1. Each partner rates their current emotional state on a scale of 1-10
2. Share what's contributing to your current emotional state
3. Identify anything you need from your partner today
4. Express appreciation for something your partner did recently
5. Plan one way you'll be kind to yourself and your partner today

This process takes about ten minutes but prevents emotional build-up and creates opportunities for support before problems become overwhelming.

The validation practice

Partners of individuals with quiet BPD often struggle to understand why "small" things trigger such intense emotional responses. The validation practice teaches both partners to focus on understanding rather than fixing emotional experiences.

Validation steps:

1. **Listen without interrupting** while your partner shares their emotional experience
2. **Reflect back what you heard** without adding your own interpretations
3. **Express understanding** of why they might feel this way given their history and current situation
4. **Ask what kind of support** they need rather than automatically offering solutions
5. **Express care for your partner** regardless of whether you understand their emotional intensity

Case example: Couple's transformation

Mark and Jennifer had been married for three years, but Mark felt like he was constantly walking on eggshells, never knowing what would upset Jennifer or how to help when she became withdrawn and distant. Jennifer felt like Mark didn't understand her and that she had to pretend to be fine to avoid burdening him.

They began practicing daily emotional temperature checks and validation exercises. Mark learned that Jennifer's withdrawal usually happened when she felt criticized or misunderstood, not when she was angry with him personally. Jennifer learned to express her needs directly rather than hoping Mark would guess what was wrong.

The breakthrough came when Jennifer was able to say, "I'm feeling really sensitive today because of stress at work. I know I might overreact to things. What I need is for you to be extra gentle with feedback and maybe give me some extra reassurance that you love me." This direct communication allowed Mark to provide appropriate support rather than guessing what Jennifer needed.

The healing power of authentic connection

Relationships that heal don't require perfection from either partner. They require honesty, patience, and willingness to grow together. For individuals with quiet BPD, these relationships provide opportunities to discover that you can be loved for your authentic self—sensitivity, struggles, and all—rather than just for your people-pleasing persona.

The process of building healing relationships is gradual and sometimes difficult. It involves taking emotional risks, tolerating vulnerability, and trusting that others can handle your complete emotional experience. But the rewards are extraordinary: relationships based on genuine connection rather than performance, love that doesn't require constant earning, and the deep satisfaction that comes from being truly known and accepted.

You deserve relationships that celebrate your sensitivity rather than requiring you to hide it, that appreciate your depth rather than asking you to be more superficial, and that support your growth rather than requiring you to stay the same. Building these relationships requires courage, but it's courage in service of one of life's most meaningful experiences—authentic human connection.

Core relationship principles

- Dating timing depends on developing enough self-knowledge and emotional stability to choose relationships from preference rather than desperation
- Disclosure about quiet BPD should happen gradually, focusing first on authentic self-expression rather than diagnostic labels
- Parenting while healing from quiet BPD requires breaking intergenerational patterns while modeling emotional authenticity and self-care
- Building supportive friendships involves showing up authentically and seeking reciprocal relationships that energize rather than drain
- Support networks should include different types of support from various people rather than expecting any single relationship to meet all needs
- Couples dealing with quiet BPD benefit from regular emotional check-ins, validation practices, and education about hidden emotional intensity

142

- Healing relationships require authenticity, patience, and mutual growth rather than perfection from either partner

Chapter 14: Career and purpose with quiet BPD

Rachel had built what looked like the perfect career—corner office, impressive title, salary that funded a comfortable lifestyle. Yet every Monday morning felt like walking toward an execution. The work itself wasn't problematic; she excelled at the analytical tasks and client relationships her role demanded. The problem was deeper: she had constructed her entire professional identity around what others expected rather than what energized her authentic self.

The transformation began during a particularly brutal performance review where her supervisor praised her "reliability" and "collaborative spirit" while suggesting she needed to be more "assertive" and "take more leadership initiative." Rachel realized she had spent eight years building a reputation for competence while systematically suppressing every aspect of her personality that felt too risky or potentially controversial. Her career success was built on performance rather than purpose, achievement rather than authenticity.

Finding meaning through activism

Rachel's breakthrough came not in another corporate strategy session, but during a community mental health awareness event where she shared her quiet BPD experiences with a small group of advocates. For the first time in her professional life, she felt energized rather than drained, passionate rather than dutiful. The conversations that followed sparked something that had been dormant for years—a sense of genuine purpose that aligned with her deepest values.

The transition from corporate success to mental health advocacy wasn't immediate or linear. Rachel spent months exploring what authentic professional engagement might look like, conducting informational interviews with people whose work inspired her, and gradually building skills in areas that genuinely excited her rather than just advancing her resume.

The purpose discovery process

Many individuals with quiet BPD struggle to identify authentic career direction because they've spent years adapting their interests to match external expectations. The process of discovering genuine purpose requires distinguishing between what you think you should want and what actually energizes you.

Values-based career exploration:

Rachel used several exercises to reconnect with her authentic professional interests:

The energy audit: She tracked which work activities energized versus drained her over several months. Tasks involving mentoring younger employees, problem-solving around team dynamics, and anything related to psychological wellness consistently appeared in her "energizing" column.

The childhood dream analysis: Looking back at her early career fantasies—teacher, counselor, writer—she identified common themes around helping others grow and communicating important information. These themes had been buried under years of practical career decisions but still resonated when she allowed herself to consider them seriously.

The jealousy investigation: She noticed which professionals triggered envy and realized these were people who combined analytical skills with advocacy work, who had platforms for sharing important messages, and who seemed to find meaning in their daily work rather than just financial success.

The impact visualization: She imagined looking back from age seventy and asking what kind of professional legacy would feel meaningful. The answer wasn't more impressive titles or higher salaries—it was having contributed to reducing stigma around mental health struggles and helping other people find their authentic voices.

Career choices that honor sensitivity

One of the most challenging aspects of career development for quiet BPD individuals involves finding professional environments that appreciate rather than penalize emotional sensitivity. Many high-functioning individuals with quiet BPD gravitate toward demanding careers that reward their perfectionist tendencies while systematically undermining their emotional well-being.

Sensitivity as professional asset

Dr. Maria Santos, a career counselor who specializes in working with highly sensitive individuals, explains that sensitivity becomes a professional liability primarily in environments that discourage emotional intelligence and authentic communication. The same traits that make quiet BPD individuals struggle in rigid corporate hierarchies can make them exceptionally effective in roles that require empathy, creativity, and emotional intelligence.

Professional environments that support sensitive individuals:

Collaborative rather than competitive cultures: Workplaces that emphasize team success over individual achievement, that encourage mentoring and knowledge sharing, and that value emotional intelligence alongside technical skills.

Mission-driven organizations: Companies or nonprofits with clear social impact missions where the work itself provides meaning and motivation beyond just financial compensation.

Creative and flexible structures: Roles that allow for autonomy, creative problem-solving, and flexible approaches to achieving outcomes rather than rigid adherence to prescribed processes.

Small to medium-sized organizations: Workplaces where individual contributions are visible and valued, where relationships matter, and where company culture can be influenced by individual employees.

146

Professional development focus: Organizations that invest in employee growth, provide training and development opportunities, and view mistakes as learning opportunities rather than performance failures.

Case example: Career transition

Michael had spent six years as a financial analyst at a large investment firm, consistently receiving positive performance reviews while experiencing increasing anxiety and emotional exhaustion. His technical skills were excellent, but the competitive environment and focus on short-term profits felt misaligned with his values and temperament.

His transition involved identifying transferable skills (analytical thinking, attention to detail, client communication) that could be applied in more suitable environments. He eventually moved to a nonprofit focused on financial literacy education, where he could use his analytical abilities while contributing to work that felt personally meaningful.

The salary reduction was significant, but Michael found that work that aligned with his values required less emotional energy to maintain, leaving him with more resources for personal relationships and self-care. His performance improved because he was no longer fighting against his natural temperament while trying to succeed professionally.

Managing perfectionism at work

Perfectionism presents a double-edged challenge for quiet BPD individuals in professional settings. The same attention to detail and high standards that can lead to excellent work quality can also create unsustainable stress, analysis paralysis, and fear of taking risks that could advance careers.

Productive vs. destructive perfectionism

Productive perfectionism:

- Focuses on continuous improvement rather than flawless performance
- Maintains perspective about which tasks require high standards versus which need "good enough" completion
- Uses mistakes as learning opportunities rather than evidence of inadequacy
- Balances quality with efficiency and deadlines
- Allows for collaboration and feedback without defensiveness

Destructive perfectionism:

- Creates paralysis around starting or finishing projects due to fear of imperfection
- Treats every task as equally critical regardless of actual importance
- Views mistakes as catastrophic failures that reflect personal inadequacy
- Prioritizes perfect work over meeting deadlines or collaborating effectively
- Prevents risk-taking or innovation due to fear of failure

Perfectionism management strategies:

The 80/20 rule: Identify which work tasks truly require 100% effort versus which would be adequately served by 80% effort. Most daily work tasks fall into the 80% category, reserving your perfectionist energy for truly high-stakes situations.

Time-boxing: Set specific time limits for projects and force yourself to submit work when the time expires, even if it feels imperfect. This prevents endless revision cycles that improve work incrementally while consuming disproportionate time and energy.

The "good enough" practice: Deliberately submit work that meets requirements without being perfect as an exercise in tolerating imperfection. Track whether the consequences are as severe as your perfectionist mind predicts (they rarely are).

Feedback reframing: View constructive criticism as information for improvement rather than evidence of failure. Practice asking clarifying questions about feedback rather than automatically assuming you've done something wrong.

Case example: Perfectionism management

Lisa, a marketing manager, spent hours crafting perfect emails to colleagues, often missing deadlines because she was still revising presentations, and avoided proposing new ideas because they might not be received positively. Her perfectionism was actually hindering her professional development rather than supporting it.

She began implementing time limits for routine tasks—thirty minutes maximum for internal emails, two hours for standard presentations, one week for project proposals. Initially, this felt terrifying because the work felt "unfinished." However, she discovered that her "imperfect" work was still well above average quality and that meeting deadlines consistently was more valuable to her career than slightly better work submitted late.

The most significant breakthrough came when she began proposing imperfect ideas during brainstorming sessions rather than waiting until she had fully developed concepts. Her colleagues appreciated her creativity and built on her initial suggestions, leading to better final outcomes than her solo perfectionist approach had achieved.

Creating sustainable success patterns

Many high-achieving individuals with quiet BPD create professional success through unsustainable patterns—excessive work hours, emotional suppression, people-pleasing, and perfectionist standards that eventually lead to burnout and career dissatisfaction. Creating sustainable success requires aligning professional achievements with personal values and emotional well-being.

The sustainability audit

149

Unsustainable success patterns:

- Working consistently longer hours than required to achieve "perfect" results
- Taking on additional responsibilities to avoid disappointing supervisors or colleagues
- Suppressing authentic opinions or ideas to maintain workplace harmony
- Using work achievements to compensate for feelings of personal inadequacy
- Avoiding vacation time or breaks due to guilt or fear of being viewed as uncommitted

Sustainable success patterns:

- Setting and maintaining boundaries around work hours and availability
- Contributing your authentic skills and perspectives rather than just being agreeable
- Taking calculated risks and learning from failures rather than avoiding all possibility of mistakes
- Finding satisfaction in the work itself rather than just external validation
- Maintaining interests and relationships outside of work that provide meaning and energy

Building sustainable patterns gradually

The transition from unsustainable to sustainable success patterns requires gradual changes rather than dramatic shifts that might jeopardize your career while you're developing new approaches.

Boundary development: Start with small boundaries—leaving work on time one day per week, not checking emails after a certain hour, or taking your full lunch break. Gradually expand these boundaries as you build confidence that your work quality and professional relationships can survive appropriate limits.

Authentic contribution: Begin sharing genuine opinions during low-stakes meetings or conversations. Volunteer for projects that align with your interests rather than just taking whatever is assigned. Gradually increase your willingness to be visible for your authentic skills and perspectives.

Risk tolerance building: Practice taking small professional risks—proposing new approaches, volunteering for challenging assignments, or speaking up during meetings. Build evidence that imperfect action often leads to better outcomes than perfectionist inaction.

From people-pleasing to authentic leadership

Many individuals with quiet BPD possess natural leadership abilities—emotional intelligence, collaborative skills, ability to see multiple perspectives—but these strengths get overshadowed by people-pleasing patterns that prevent authentic leadership development.

The people-pleasing leadership trap

Traditional people-pleasing patterns make individuals appear to be team players but prevent them from developing the assertiveness, decision-making ability, and authentic vision that true leadership requires. People-pleasers often get passed over for leadership roles because they're seen as followers rather than leaders, despite possessing many qualities that would make them effective managers.

Authentic leadership development:

Vision development: Identify what you believe needs to change or improve in your workplace or field. Authentic leadership begins with having opinions about how things could be better rather than just adapting to current conditions.

Decision-making practice: Volunteer for roles that require making decisions, even small ones. Practice tolerating the discomfort of making choices that not everyone will agree with.

Conflict navigation: Learn to address disagreements directly rather than avoiding them or automatically accommodating others' preferences. This doesn't mean becoming argumentative—it means being willing to engage in respectful disagreement when necessary.

Authentic communication: Practice expressing your genuine thoughts and opinions during meetings and conversations rather than just agreeing with whatever seems most acceptable.

Team advocacy: Learn to advocate for your team's needs, resources, and recognition rather than just managing up by telling supervisors what they want to hear.

Case example: Leadership development

David had been in the same mid-level position for five years despite consistently positive performance reviews. His supervisors valued his reliability and collaborative spirit but never considered him for promotion to management roles. He realized that his people-pleasing patterns made him appear passive rather than leadership material.

His development process involved gradually taking more visible positions on workplace issues. He began advocating for process improvements he genuinely believed would help the team, volunteering to lead projects that interested him, and expressing opinions during strategic planning meetings.

The breakthrough came when he proposed a new client communication system that he had been thinking about for months but had never suggested. His initiative impressed supervisors who hadn't realized he had strategic ideas beyond just implementing others' decisions. Within six months, he was promoted to team lead and discovered that leadership felt energizing rather than draining when it was based on authentic engagement rather than people-pleasing performance.

Professional development and workplace wellness

Career satisfaction for individuals with quiet BPD often depends more on workplace emotional climate than on salary or title. Creating professional environments that support rather than undermine emotional well-being requires both individual advocacy and strategic career choices.

Workplace wellness strategies:

Energy management: Identify which work activities and interactions energize versus drain you. Advocate for role responsibilities that play to your strengths while minimizing energy-depleting tasks when possible.

Relationship building: Cultivate authentic professional relationships with colleagues who appreciate your genuine contributions rather than just your people-pleasing persona.

Boundary maintenance: Develop and communicate clear boundaries around availability, work methods, and interaction styles that support your emotional well-being.

Professional development: Pursue training and development opportunities that align with your authentic interests and career direction rather than just what seems most impressive on a resume.

Stress management: Build workplace stress management strategies that work with your temperament rather than against it—this might include scheduled breaks, quiet workspace arrangements, or flexible scheduling when possible.

Self-advocacy: Practice communicating your needs, accomplishments, and career goals directly rather than hoping supervisors will notice your contributions automatically.

Creating meaning in any role

While finding the perfect job that aligns completely with your values and temperament is ideal, it's not always immediately possible. In the meantime, you can create meaning and satisfaction in imperfect roles by:

Identifying opportunities to help others: Even in roles that don't feel personally meaningful, you can often find ways to mentor colleagues, improve team dynamics, or contribute to workplace culture in positive ways.

Developing transferable skills: Use current roles to build skills that will support your longer-term career goals, even if the current position isn't your dream job.

Maintaining perspective: View current roles as stepping stones rather than permanent situations, while still engaging fully in your current responsibilities.

Building professional networks: Use current positions to meet people and learn about opportunities that might be more aligned with your authentic interests and values.

The goal isn't to find perfect work immediately, but to gradually move toward professional environments and roles that appreciate your authentic strengths while providing the meaning and satisfaction that make daily work feel like contribution rather than obligation.

Professional wisdom gained

Career fulfillment for individuals with quiet BPD comes not from achieving traditional markers of success, but from finding roles that honor your sensitivity, align with your values, and allow you to contribute your authentic strengths rather than just your people-pleasing persona. This often requires courage to make changes that prioritize meaning over money, authenticity over approval, and sustainable satisfaction over unsustainable achievement.

The professional journey may involve taking risks, accepting lower salaries, or disappointing people who preferred your accommodating previous self. But the rewards—work that energizes rather than drains, colleagues who appreciate your genuine contributions, and the deep satisfaction that comes from authentic professional engagement—make the challenges worthwhile.

You deserve work that celebrates your sensitivity rather than requiring you to suppress it, that appreciates your emotional intelligence rather than viewing it as weakness, and that provides opportunities to contribute meaningfully rather than just perform successfully.

Key professional insights

- Career satisfaction for quiet BPD individuals comes from aligning work with authentic values rather than just achieving external markers of success
- Professional environments that honor sensitivity include collaborative cultures, mission-driven organizations, and flexible structures that value emotional intelligence
- Managing workplace perfectionism requires distinguishing between tasks that need high standards versus those that need "good enough" completion
- Sustainable success patterns involve setting boundaries, contributing authentically, and taking calculated risks rather than people-pleasing and perfectionist overwork
- Leadership development requires moving from people-pleasing patterns to authentic vision, decision-making, and willingness to engage in respectful conflict
- Workplace wellness depends on energy management, boundary maintenance, authentic relationship building, and strategic self-advocacy
- Career meaning can be created in imperfect roles through helping others, skill development, and maintaining perspective about longer-term goals

Chapter 15: Crisis planning for invisible emergencies

The text message arrived at 2:17 AM on a Tuesday: "Are you okay? I had a weird feeling you might need someone to check in." Lisa stared at her phone in the darkness of her bedroom, tears streaming down her face. For the past three hours, she had been sitting with a bottle of prescription medications, not planning to take them, but finding strange comfort in knowing they were there—a potential escape if the emotional pain became truly unbearable.

Her friend's message broke the spell. Someone had sensed her distress despite her perfect facade at work that day, her cheerful social media posts, and her carefully maintained appearance of having everything together. This moment of connection reminded Lisa that her pain was real even when invisible, that her struggles mattered even when hidden, and that she deserved support even when she looked fine from the outside.

Crisis planning for quiet BPD involves preparing for emotional emergencies that others can't see—moments when internal emotional storms become so intense that normal coping strategies feel insufficient. These aren't dramatic crises with obvious warning signs; they're invisible emergencies that can escalate quickly and require specific safety strategies designed for people who suffer in silence.

Recognizing your unique warning signs

Traditional crisis intervention focuses on obvious signs—behavioral changes, verbal threats, visible self-harm. Quiet BPD crises often lack these external markers, making early recognition challenging for both the individual and their support system. Learning to identify your personal early warning signs can prevent emotional overwhelm from escalating to dangerous levels.

Internal warning signs that others can't see:

Emotional numbness escalation: Moving from normal emotional suppression to complete inability to feel anything—positive or negative emotions become equally inaccessible, creating a sense of being disconnected from your own life.

Perfectionist paralysis intensification: Normal high standards become impossible standards that prevent starting or completing any tasks. You might spend hours staring at blank documents or emails, unable to write anything because nothing feels adequate.

Social mask exhaustion: The energy required to maintain your composed exterior becomes overwhelming. Simple social interactions that usually feel manageable begin requiring tremendous effort, and you start avoiding people because you can't maintain the performance.

Identity dissolution experiences: Normal identity uncertainty becomes acute confusion about who you are or what's real about your personality. You might feel like you're completely fake or that there's no authentic self underneath your various social personas.

Abandonment sensitivity amplification: Normal fears about relationships escalate to constant vigilance for signs of rejection. You might interpret neutral expressions as evidence of disapproval or analyze text messages for hidden meanings that suggest people are pulling away.

Case example: Early warning recognition

Marcus learned to recognize his crisis pattern through careful observation over several months. His early warning signs included: difficulty making simple decisions (what to eat, what to wear), increased irritability at work despite maintaining professional demeanor, sleeping more than usual while still feeling exhausted, and finding no enjoyment in activities that normally brought pleasure.

The key insight was recognizing that these signs appeared 3-5 days before his emotional state became genuinely dangerous. This gave him a window for intervention—reaching out to his therapist, implementing extra self-care strategies, and alerting trusted friends that he might need additional support.

Physical warning signs that accompany emotional crises:

Quiet BPD crises often include physical symptoms that might be dismissed as stress or minor health issues:

- **Sleep disturbances**: Sleeping much more or less than usual, or sleeping but not feeling rested
- **Appetite changes**: Complete loss of appetite or compulsive eating without awareness of hunger/fullness
- **Physical tension**: Chronic headaches, jaw clenching, shoulder tension that doesn't respond to normal relaxation techniques
- **Digestive issues**: Nausea, stomach pain, or digestive problems that worsen during emotional stress
- **Fatigue**: Exhaustion that rest doesn't improve, feeling like you're moving through thick fog
- **Sensory sensitivity**: Increased sensitivity to lights, sounds, or textures that normally don't bother you

Behavioral warning signs that might be subtle:

- **Routine disruption**: Abandoning self-care practices, letting household tasks accumulate, or missing appointments you normally keep
- **Social withdrawal**: Declining invitations, taking longer to respond to messages, or avoiding phone calls
- **Work performance changes**: Making more mistakes, having difficulty concentrating, or avoiding challenging tasks
- **Emotional eating or restriction**: Using food to cope with emotions in ways that feel different from your normal eating patterns
- **Technology overuse or avoidance**: Spending excessive time scrolling social media or completely avoiding electronic communication

Safety planning for internalized self-harm

Traditional safety planning focuses on preventing external self-harm behaviors—cutting, overdoses, or other visible forms of self-injury. Quiet BPD safety planning must address internalized forms of self-harm that can be equally dangerous but remain invisible to others.

Internal self-harm behaviors common in quiet BPD:

Emotional self-punishment: Deliberately dwelling on painful memories, engaging in harsh self-criticism, or ruminating on perceived failures as a form of self-inflicted emotional pain.

Social self-isolation: Withdrawing from supportive relationships as punishment for being "too much" or "too needy," creating additional emotional pain through loneliness.

Opportunity sabotage: Avoiding positive experiences, declining invitations, or undermining your own success because you believe you don't deserve good things.

Sleep deprivation: Staying awake as self-punishment or to avoid dreams, creating physical and emotional exhaustion that worsens mental health symptoms.

Neglecting basic needs: Skipping meals, avoiding medical care, or neglecting personal hygiene as forms of self-punishment that feel less obvious than direct self-harm.

Perfectionist self-torture: Setting impossible standards and then criticizing yourself harshly when you inevitably fall short, creating cycles of achievement pressure and failure-based self-attack.

Creating a safety plan for invisible crises:

Step 1: Early warning sign checklist Create a written list of your personal warning signs and check it weekly during stable periods, daily during stressful times. Include physical, emotional, and behavioral indicators that typically appear before crises escalate.

Step 2: Internal self-soothing strategies Develop a toolkit of activities that can interrupt internal self-harm patterns:

- **Grounding techniques** that work when you're alone (5-4-3-2-1 sensory awareness, holding ice cubes, intense physical exercise)
- **Self-compassion phrases** that counter harsh self-criticism ("This is temporary," "I'm doing the best I can right now," "I deserve kindness during difficult times")
- **Distraction activities** that require enough mental engagement to interrupt rumination cycles (puzzles, detailed creative projects, learning new skills)

Step 3: External connection protocols Identify specific people you can contact during different levels of crisis and plan exactly how you'll reach out:

- **Level 1** (early warning signs): Text or email check-in with 2-3 trusted people
- **Level 2** (moderate crisis): Phone call or video chat with someone who understands your struggles
- **Level 3** (severe crisis): Immediate in-person support or professional crisis intervention

Step 4: Environmental safety modifications Make your physical environment safer during emotional crises:

- Remove or secure items that could be used for self-harm
- Create comfort spaces with soft lighting, comforting objects, and calming sensory input
- Prepare care packages for difficult times (comfort foods, soft blankets, inspiring books or music)
- Establish technology boundaries (apps that limit social media during vulnerable times, phones that filter negative content)

Case example: Internal safety planning

Jennifer created a safety plan after recognizing that her crises involved emotional self-harm rather than physical self-injury. Her plan included:

Early warning signs: Difficulty making decisions, sleeping more than 10 hours per day, avoiding texts from friends, and losing interest in her normally enjoyable photography hobby.

Self-soothing toolkit: Taking hot baths with specific essential oils, doing jigsaw puzzles, listening to particular playlists that felt comforting without being overly emotional, and practicing progressive muscle relaxation.

Connection plan: Texting her sister during level 1 warnings, calling her therapist or best friend during level 2 crises, and having her sister come stay with her during level 3 emergencies.

Environmental modifications: Removing alcohol from her apartment during stressful periods, preparing frozen meals in advance so she could eat without decision-making energy, and setting her phone to airplane mode during evening hours when rumination typically intensified.

Recognizing when professional help is needed

One of the most challenging aspects of quiet BPD crises involves knowing when to seek professional help. The absence of dramatic external symptoms can make it difficult to gauge when emotional distress has reached levels that require clinical intervention rather than self-help strategies.

Indicators that professional help is needed:

Persistent inability to function: When basic daily tasks—showering, eating, working, sleeping—become consistently difficult for more than a few days despite your best self-care efforts.

Escalating self-harm thoughts: When thoughts about self-punishment become more frequent, specific, or appealing, even if you're not planning to act on them immediately.

Complete emotional numbness: When you can't access any emotions—positive or negative—for extended periods, feeling like you're living in a gray fog without connection to your own experience.

Relationship withdrawal: When you isolate completely from all social connections for more than a week, especially if this isolation feels protective but also scary.

Suicidal ideation: Any thoughts about death or suicide, even passive ones like "I wish I could just disappear" or "Everyone would be better off without me."

Substance use escalation: Using alcohol, prescription medications, or other substances to manage emotions in ways that feel different from your normal use patterns.

Reality distortion: Questioning what's real about your experiences, relationships, or identity to the extent that you feel disconnected from reality.

Case example: Professional help recognition

Michael had been managing his quiet BPD symptoms independently for months using therapy skills and self-care strategies. However, during a particularly stressful period at work, he began experiencing persistent thoughts about disappearing—not suicide exactly, but fantasies about leaving his life entirely and starting over somewhere no one knew him.

Initially, he dismissed these thoughts as normal stress responses. But when he realized he had spent several hours researching how to disappear completely and had begun viewing these fantasies as genuinely appealing rather than just temporary escape wishes, he recognized that his crisis had escalated beyond self-help capacity.

162

He contacted his therapist for an emergency appointment and discovered that his thoughts about disappearing were actually a form of suicidal ideation—psychological escape rather than physical suicide, but equally concerning. Professional intervention helped him develop specific strategies for managing these thoughts while addressing the underlying stressors that had triggered the crisis.

Building your crisis response team

Effective crisis support for quiet BPD requires people who understand that serious emotional distress can exist without obvious external symptoms. Your crisis response team needs to include individuals who can recognize subtle signs of distress and respond appropriately to invisible emergencies.

Team member characteristics:

Emotional availability: People who can be reached during non-business hours and who understand that emotional crises don't follow convenient schedules.

Distress recognition skills: Individuals who know you well enough to notice when something is wrong, even when you're maintaining your composed exterior.

Non-judgmental support: People who won't minimize your struggles or suggest that you should be able to handle things independently just because you appear high-functioning.

Practical assistance capability: Team members who can provide concrete help—transportation to appointments, companionship during difficult times, or assistance with daily tasks when you're overwhelmed.

Professional boundary respect: Understanding the difference between peer support and professional intervention, and knowing when to encourage professional help rather than trying to provide therapy.

163

Different types of crisis support needed:

Immediate emotional support: Someone who can provide comfort and connection during acute emotional distress, available for phone calls or in-person visits during crises.

Practical crisis management: People who can help with concrete needs—driving you to appointments, staying with you overnight, or managing work/family responsibilities when you're unable to function normally.

Professional liaison: Someone who can communicate with your therapist, doctor, or other professionals if you become unable to advocate for yourself during severe crises.

Long-term stability support: Individuals who can provide ongoing check-ins and support during recovery periods, helping you rebuild functioning after crises resolve.

Case example: Crisis team development

After experiencing a serious emotional crisis that left her unable to work for several days, Rebecca realized she needed a more structured support system. She identified:

Sister (immediate emotional support): Could be reached at any time, understood Rebecca's struggles with anxiety and depression, and lived close enough to provide in-person support when needed.

Best friend (practical crisis management): Had offered to help during difficult times, could provide childcare for Rebecca's daughter, and was comfortable staying overnight during crises.

Therapist (professional liaison): Had emergency contact protocols, could provide crisis appointments, and could coordinate with other healthcare providers if needed.

Neighbor (long-term stability support): Reliable for daily check-ins, could help with routine tasks like grocery shopping, and was available for low-key companionship during recovery periods.

Rebecca practiced reaching out to each team member during non-crisis times, establishing communication patterns and clarifying what types of support each person could provide. This preparation made it easier to ask for help during actual emergencies.

Crisis toolkit development

Having specific tools and resources prepared in advance can make the difference between manageable emotional distress and escalated crises. Your crisis toolkit should include items that work specifically for your patterns of emotional dysregulation and can be accessed quickly when your ability to think clearly is compromised.

Physical comfort items:

- **Weighted blanket or heavy comforter** for grounding during dissociation or emotional numbness
- **Comfort foods** that are easy to prepare and don't require decision-making energy
- **Sensory items** like soft textures, pleasant scents, or calming music playlists
- **Temperature regulation tools** like heating pads, ice packs, or materials for warm baths
- **Emergency medication** if prescribed by healthcare providers for crisis situations

Communication tools:

- **Pre-written text messages** for reaching out when you can't find words to explain what's wrong
- **Contact list** with phone numbers easily accessible even if your phone is dead or lost
- **Crisis hotline numbers** programmed into your phone and written in multiple locations

- **Apps** designed for mental health crisis support, with accounts set up in advance

Self-care supplies:

- **Hygiene essentials** prepared in easy-to-access locations for times when basic self-care feels overwhelming
- **Medication organizers** to prevent confusion about what you've taken during crisis periods
- **Prepared meals** that require minimal preparation and provide adequate nutrition
- **Sleep aids** like blackout curtains, comfortable pillows, or white noise machines

Information resources:

- **Crisis plan copies** in multiple locations—your home, car, work, and with trusted support people
- **Medical information** including medication lists, healthcare provider contact information, and relevant medical conditions
- **Insurance and legal documents** easily accessible in case crisis requires professional intervention

The goal isn't to have everything you might possibly need, but to prepare specific tools that address your particular crisis patterns and can be accessed quickly when your cognitive functioning is impaired by emotional distress.

Professional resources and emergency protocols

Knowing when and how to access professional crisis support can prevent emotional emergencies from escalating to life-threatening levels. This requires understanding different levels of professional intervention and having contact information readily available.

Levels of professional crisis support:

Therapist emergency contact: Most therapists provide some form of crisis contact for established clients. Clarify with your therapist what constitutes an appropriate emergency contact and how to reach them outside normal business hours.

Crisis hotlines: National and local crisis lines provide immediate phone support from trained counselors. These services are confidential, available 24/7, and designed specifically for emotional emergencies.

Crisis mobile teams: Some areas have mobile crisis response teams that can provide in-person evaluation and support in your home rather than requiring emergency room visits.

Emergency room evaluation: For severe crises involving safety concerns, emergency rooms can provide immediate assessment and referral to appropriate mental health services.

Psychiatric urgent care: Some areas have psychiatric urgent care facilities that provide specialized mental health crisis intervention in less intensive settings than emergency rooms.

Hospital admission: For crises that pose immediate safety risks or involve complete inability to function, voluntary or involuntary hospital admission may be necessary for stabilization and intensive treatment.

Understanding these options in advance and having contact information readily available can help you or your support team make appropriate decisions during crisis situations when clear thinking is compromised.

Emergency preparedness

Crisis planning for quiet BPD requires accepting that emotional emergencies are possible even when you generally function well and appear stable to others. Preparation doesn't mean expecting crises to occur—it means reducing the barriers to getting help if crises do develop.

The most important aspect of crisis planning involves giving yourself permission to seek help even when you "look fine" to others, even when you feel like you should be able to handle difficulties independently, and even when you worry about burdening others with your struggles. Your internal emotional experience is valid regardless of your external appearance, and you deserve support during difficult times regardless of how well you function in other areas of your life.

Crisis preparation is an act of self-compassion—acknowledging your vulnerabilities while taking concrete steps to ensure your safety. It's planning for the possibility that your coping strategies might temporarily become insufficient, while building systems that can support you until your normal functioning returns.

Emergency planning essentials

- Early warning signs for quiet BPD crises are often internal and invisible to others, requiring careful self-monitoring and documentation
- Safety planning must address internalized self-harm behaviors like emotional self-punishment, social isolation, and opportunity sabotage
- Professional help indicators include persistent dysfunction, escalating self-harm thoughts, complete numbness, relationship withdrawal, and any suicidal ideation
- Crisis response teams need members who can recognize subtle distress, provide emotional and practical support, and respect professional boundaries
- Crisis toolkits should include physical comfort items, communication tools, self-care supplies, and information resources prepared in advance
- Professional crisis resources range from therapist emergency contact to crisis hotlines, mobile teams, urgent care, and hospital admission depending on severity

- Effective crisis planning requires accepting that emotional emergencies can occur despite general high functioning and external appearance of stability

Chapter 16: A guide for families and loved ones

Living with someone who has quiet BPD presents unique challenges that most families never see coming. Your loved one might appear composed, successful, and perfectly fine to the outside world, while privately struggling with intense emotional pain that remains largely invisible. This disconnect between public persona and private suffering often leaves family members confused, frustrated, and unsure how to help.

The person you care about has likely mastered the art of emotional concealment. They smile at family gatherings while internally battling overwhelming shame. They excel at work while secretly believing they're frauds who don't deserve success. They maintain friendships while feeling fundamentally disconnected from others. This emotional camouflage serves as both protection and prison, keeping their pain hidden while preventing authentic connection.

Understanding this hidden struggle requires a fundamental shift in how you perceive mental health. Unlike more obvious conditions that display clear symptoms, quiet BPD operates beneath the surface. Your loved one isn't being dramatic or attention-seeking – they're working overtime to appear normal while managing intense internal chaos.

Understanding the Invisible: When your loved one seems fine but isn't

Sarah's mother knew something was wrong, but she couldn't pinpoint exactly what. Her 28-year-old daughter had a successful marketing career, lived in a beautiful apartment, and maintained an active social media presence filled with smiling photos. Yet during family visits, Sarah seemed distant and exhausted. She would excuse herself frequently to "check work emails" but her mother noticed she often returned with red-rimmed eyes.

The invisibility of quiet BPD symptoms creates a particular burden for families. Traditional signs of mental health struggles – dramatic outbursts, obvious self-harm, or social withdrawal – aren't present. Instead, you might notice:

Perfectionist behavior that seems excessive. Your loved one cannot tolerate making mistakes and becomes disproportionately upset over minor errors. They might spend hours redoing projects that already meet requirements or become paralyzed when faced with tasks they cannot execute perfectly.

Physical complaints without clear medical causes. Chronic headaches, stomach issues, or fatigue that doctors cannot fully explain often accompany the emotional stress of quiet BPD. Your loved one might frequently visit medical professionals seeking answers for symptoms that stem from internal emotional turmoil.

Subtle withdrawal from emotional intimacy. They participate in family activities but seem emotionally absent. They answer questions about their lives with surface-level responses and redirect conversations away from personal topics. This emotional distancing protects them from vulnerability but creates a sense of disconnection within relationships.

Overcommitment followed by exhaustion. They say yes to every request, volunteer for additional responsibilities, and maintain packed schedules. This pattern often leads to burnout, which they interpret as personal failure rather than natural consequences of overextension.

Michael's father noticed these patterns during weekly family dinners. Michael would arrive looking polished and professional, engage in pleasant conversation, and help with cleanup. However, he never shared genuine struggles or celebrated personal victories. When his father asked direct questions about Michael's wellbeing, he received standard responses: "Everything's fine," "Work's going well," or "Nothing new to report."

171

The challenge for families lies in recognizing distress signals that your loved one has learned to mask effectively. They've developed sophisticated coping mechanisms that maintain functional appearances while preventing others from seeing their internal struggles.

Recognizing subtle distress signals

Learning to identify hidden distress requires developing sensitivity to subtle behavioral and emotional shifts. Your loved one won't announce their struggles, so you must become skilled at reading between the lines.

Changes in communication patterns often provide the first clues. Someone who typically responds to text messages immediately might begin taking hours or days to reply. Their responses might become shorter, more formal, or lack their usual warmth. Phone conversations that once flowed naturally might feel stilted or rushed.

Lisa's sister noticed this pattern during a particularly difficult period. Lisa, who normally sent lengthy, detailed texts about her day, began responding with single words or thumbs-up emojis. When her sister called, Lisa would cut conversations short, claiming she needed to handle "urgent" tasks that seemed to multiply whenever emotional topics arose.

Sleep and eating patterns frequently reflect internal distress. Your loved one might mention sleeping too much or too little, eating irregularly, or losing interest in foods they previously enjoyed. They might make casual comments about being "too busy to eat properly" or "not sleeping well lately" without acknowledging these as symptoms of deeper struggles.

Social behavior changes can be particularly revealing. Someone who typically accepts social invitations might begin declining without clear explanations. They might attend events but leave early or seem disconnected during interactions. Alternatively, they might increase social activities to dangerous levels, using constant busyness to avoid internal reflection.

David's wife observed this pattern when he began accepting every social invitation they received while simultaneously seeming exhausted and overwhelmed. He would return from events claiming they were "fine" but would spend the following day in bed, claiming he needed to "catch up on rest."

Emotional regulation difficulties manifest in subtle ways. Your loved one might become unusually irritated by minor inconveniences, struggle to recover from small disappointments, or seem emotionally flat during typically exciting events. They might apologize excessively for normal human mistakes or reactions.

Physical presentation changes can signal internal distress. Your loved one might begin neglecting self-care routines they previously maintained, such as regular exercise, skincare, or grooming habits. Alternatively, they might become obsessive about appearance, spending excessive time and money on looking perfect.

The key to recognizing these signals lies in understanding your loved one's baseline behavior and noting deviations from their normal patterns. Someone who typically maintains impeccable appearance suddenly wearing wrinkled clothes might be struggling as much as someone who typically dresses casually suddenly becoming obsessive about fashion.

Validation without enabling

Responding appropriately to quiet BPD requires mastering the delicate balance between validation and enabling. Your loved one needs acknowledgment of their struggles without reinforcement of unhealthy coping mechanisms or rescue behaviors that prevent growth.

Validation acknowledges emotional reality without solving problems. When your loved one mentions feeling overwhelmed at work, validation might sound like: "That sounds really stressful. You've been handling a lot lately." This response acknowledges their experience without offering solutions, advice, or minimization.

Enabling, by contrast, might involve calling their boss to explain their absence, completing their responsibilities, or offering constant reassurance that reinforces their need for external validation. While these responses come from love, they prevent your loved one from developing internal coping skills and self-reliance.

Jennifer's parents learned this distinction through trial and error. Initially, when Jennifer expressed anxiety about work presentations, they would spend hours helping her practice, reviewing her materials, and offering extensive reassurance. This pattern escalated until Jennifer required their involvement for increasingly minor work tasks.

With professional guidance, they learned to validate her anxiety ("Presentations can definitely feel nerve-wracking") while encouraging her capability ("You've handled challenging presentations successfully before"). They stopped providing extensive help while remaining emotionally supportive.

Emotional validation focuses on feelings rather than fixing. Your loved one might share feelings of inadequacy, failure, or overwhelm. Validation acknowledges these emotions as understandable given their circumstances, without rushing to contradict or correct their perceptions.

For example, when your loved one says, "I feel like I'm failing at everything," validation might respond: "You're going through a really tough time right now. These feelings make sense given what you're dealing with." This acknowledges their emotional experience without arguing against their perspective or offering immediate solutions.

Avoid validation that reinforces negative self-concepts. While acknowledging their emotional pain, avoid agreeing with harsh self-criticism or catastrophic thinking patterns. You can validate their emotional experience without confirming destructive beliefs about themselves or their capabilities.

If your loved one says, "I'm such a burden to everyone," validation might sound like: "You're clearly struggling right now, and that's really painful" rather than "You're not a burden" (which dismisses their feeling) or "Everyone does feel burdened sometimes" (which confirms their fear).

Set clear boundaries around rescue behaviors. Loving someone with quiet BPD often triggers impulses to shield them from consequences or solve their problems. While these impulses stem from care, acting on them prevents your loved one from developing resilience and problem-solving skills.

This might mean allowing them to experience natural consequences of overcommitment, such as fatigue or missed opportunities, without stepping in to fix situations they created. It might mean listening to their work stress without offering to intervene with their employer or complete their tasks.

Setting loving boundaries

Boundaries protect both you and your loved one from unhealthy relationship dynamics while maintaining connection and support. People with quiet BPD often struggle with boundaries themselves – they might have difficulty saying no, setting limits, or recognizing their own needs. This makes it essential for family members to model healthy boundary-setting.

Establish clear limits on emotional labor. Your loved one might rely heavily on family members for emotional regulation, seeking constant reassurance, lengthy processing conversations, or rescue from difficult situations. While offering support is natural, unlimited availability can create unhealthy dependence and exhaust your emotional resources.

Healthy boundaries might include designated times for processing conversations, limits on crisis calls, or agreements about problem-solving versus venting sessions. These boundaries aren't punitive – they're protective structures that maintain sustainable relationships.

Tom's mother implemented this boundary after months of nightly calls that lasted two to three hours. She loved her son and wanted to support him, but these conversations were affecting her sleep, work performance, and relationship with her husband. She established a boundary that processing calls would be limited to one hour and would not occur after 9 PM unless there was a genuine emergency.

Initially, Tom felt rejected and accused his mother of not caring about his struggles. However, with consistent, loving enforcement of this boundary, their conversations became more focused and productive. Tom began developing other coping strategies and their relationship improved.

Maintain your own emotional wellbeing. Loving someone with quiet BPD can be emotionally draining, particularly because their struggles often remain invisible to others. You might feel like you're the only one who truly understands their pain, creating pressure to be constantly available and supportive.

This dynamic is unsustainable and ultimately unhelpful. Your loved one needs to see healthy emotional regulation modeled, not anxious caretaking. They need relationships with people who maintain their own wellbeing, not relationships where their struggles dominate all interactions.

Create structure around helping behaviors. Decide in advance what types of help you're willing to provide and under what circumstances. This prevents reactive decision-making during crisis moments when your loved one's distress might override your better judgment.

For example, you might decide you're willing to provide emotional support and encouragement but not financial rescue or completion of their responsibilities. You might agree to help with practical tasks during genuine emergencies but not during situations they created through poor planning or overcommitment.

Communicate boundaries with compassion. Boundary-setting conversations should emphasize your care for your loved one while clearly stating your limits. The message should be: "I love you and I'm limiting my availability to maintain my ability to support you long-term."

Boundaries aren't ultimatums or punishments – they're loving limits that protect relationships from becoming unsustainable. Frame boundaries as investments in your relationship's longevity rather than restrictions on your love or support.

Managing your own emotional health

Supporting someone with quiet BPD requires intentional attention to your own emotional wellbeing. The invisible nature of their struggles can create chronic stress for family members who recognize the depth of their loved one's pain while watching them maintain successful external appearances.

Acknowledge the unique stress of invisible illness. Traditional support systems often fail to understand the challenges of loving someone whose mental health struggles aren't obvious. Friends and extended family might not understand why you're concerned about someone who appears successful and functional.

This isolation can compound your stress and create doubt about your perceptions. You might question whether your loved one is truly struggling or whether you're overreacting to normal life stress. Trust your observations and seek support from mental health professionals or support groups familiar with quiet BPD.

Develop your own support network. Identify people you can talk to honestly about your experiences without betraying your loved one's privacy. This might include therapists, support groups, or trusted friends who understand mental health challenges.

Having support is not disloyal to your loved one – it's essential for maintaining your capacity to be helpful. You cannot provide steady support if you're emotionally depleted or isolated in your concern.

Practice emotional detachment. Learn to separate your emotional wellbeing from your loved one's daily struggles. Their bad days don't need to become your bad days. Their progress or setbacks don't need to determine your mood or self-worth.

This detachment isn't coldness – it's healthy differentiation that allows you to remain supportive without becoming emotionally consumed by their journey. You can care deeply while maintaining emotional stability that doesn't fluctuate with their daily experiences.

Maintain your own interests and relationships. Don't allow concern for your loved one to consume all your emotional energy or social time. Continue pursuing activities you enjoy, maintaining other relationships, and investing in your own growth and development.

Your loved one benefits more from relationships with people who have rich, fulfilling lives than from relationships with people whose entire focus centers on their struggles. Model the balanced life you hope they'll eventually create for themselves.

Set realistic expectations for change. Recovery from quiet BPD typically involves gradual progress with occasional setbacks rather than steady, linear improvement. Understanding this reality helps prevent disappointment and maintains hope during difficult periods.

Your love and support matter tremendously, but they cannot cure your loved one's condition or control their choices. Accept your influence while releasing responsibility for outcomes beyond your control.

Family Stories: Lessons from the journey

The Martinez family discovered their daughter Elena's quiet BPD diagnosis during her junior year of college, though they recognized in hindsight that signs had been present for years. Elena had always been the "easy" child – studious, compliant, and seemingly self-sufficient compared to her more dramatic younger brother.

The revelation came during Elena's hospitalization following what appeared to be a stress-related breakdown. She had been maintaining a 4.0 GPA while working part-time, volunteering, and participating in three campus organizations. To everyone's surprise, she had also been secretly struggling with severe depression, anxiety, and suicidal thoughts for over two years.

Elena's mother, Rosa, initially blamed herself for missing the signs. "How could I not know my own daughter was suffering so much?" she asked repeatedly during family therapy sessions. The therapist helped Rosa understand that Elena's symptoms were designed to be invisible and that even trained professionals often miss quiet BPD presentations.

The family learned to recognize Elena's subtle distress signals and respond supportively without enabling her perfectionist tendencies. They created new family traditions that emphasized connection over achievement and established regular check-ins that focused on emotional wellbeing rather than academic or career success.

Two years later, Elena credits her family's support as crucial to her recovery. However, she emphasizes that their willingness to set boundaries and maintain their own lives prevented her from becoming overly dependent on their emotional regulation.

The Chen family faced different challenges when their son David's quiet BPD symptoms emerged during a career transition in his early thirties. David had always been successful professionally, but changing jobs triggered intense identity confusion and emotional instability that he kept carefully hidden from colleagues and most friends.

David's parents noticed changes during their weekly family dinners. He became increasingly quiet, seemed exhausted despite his usual professional success, and began declining social invitations he would typically accept. When they expressed concern, David insisted everything was fine and became irritated by their questions.

The family spent months walking on eggshells, unsure how to address their concerns without pushing David further away. They eventually sought guidance from a therapist specializing in family dynamics and quiet BPD, who helped them understand how to express care without being intrusive.

They learned to make observations rather than accusations ("You seem tired lately" rather than "Something's wrong with you") and to offer specific support rather than general help ("I'm free Saturday if you want company grocery shopping" rather than "Let me know if you need anything").

David initially resisted their efforts but gradually began accepting small offers of support. He eventually sought therapy independently and credits his family's patient, non-judgmental approach with helping him feel safe enough to address his struggles.

The Williams family's journey began when their daughter Ashley's college roommate contacted them with concerns about Ashley's behavior. The roommate reported that Ashley spent most evenings alone in her room, rarely ate meals with others, and seemed to study obsessively despite earning excellent grades.

Ashley's parents were shocked by this description, as she presented herself as happy and socially engaged during their phone conversations. When they visited campus, Ashley maintained her cheerful facade but they noticed signs of exhaustion and weight loss she had managed to hide during video calls.

The family's initial attempts to address their concerns backfired. Ashley became defensive and accused them of not trusting her independence. She threatened to stop communicating with them entirely if they continued "interfering" in her life.

Through family therapy, the Williams learned to approach Ashley's struggles indirectly. Instead of confronting her about specific behaviors, they focused on strengthening their relationship and creating safe spaces for her to share if she chose to do so.

They began sending care packages focused on comfort rather than nutrition (which Ashley interpreted as criticism of her eating habits). They shared their own struggles and vulnerabilities during phone calls, modeling emotional openness without demanding reciprocity.

Over time, Ashley began sharing small pieces of her experience. She eventually disclosed her struggles with perfectionism and social anxiety, leading to her decision to seek counseling. The key breakthrough came when her parents demonstrated they could handle her imperfections without trying to fix them immediately.

Understanding quiet BPD as a family member requires patience, education, and commitment to your own wellbeing. Your loved one's recovery journey benefits most from relationships that provide steady support without enabling unhealthy patterns or sacrificing your own emotional health.

The invisibility of quiet BPD symptoms challenges traditional approaches to supporting someone with mental illness. Your loved one isn't seeking attention or being dramatic – they're managing intense internal experiences while maintaining functional external appearances. This requires recognition, validation, and support that acknowledges their hidden struggles.

Your role involves learning new skills in recognition, validation, boundary-setting, and self-care. These skills benefit not only your relationship with your loved one but also your overall approach to healthy relationships and emotional wellbeing.

Key Takeaways for Supporting Your Loved One:

- Learn to recognize subtle distress signals that your loved one has mastered hiding from the outside world
- Validate their emotional experiences without enabling unhealthy coping mechanisms or rescue behaviors
- Set loving boundaries that protect both your wellbeing and theirs from unsustainable relationship dynamics

- Maintain your own emotional health through support networks, interests, and realistic expectations for change
- Trust your observations while seeking professional guidance to understand how best to help
- Remember that your love and support matter tremendously, even when progress seems slow or invisible

Chapter 17: Professional guidance for treating quiet BPD

The clinical presentation of quiet BPD poses unique challenges that require specialized assessment strategies and treatment approaches. Traditional diagnostic frameworks often miss these clients, who present as high-functioning individuals with subtle symptomatology that doesn't align with classic BPD presentations. Mental health professionals must develop sensitivity to hidden presentations while adapting evidence-based treatments for clients who internalize rather than externalize their emotional dysregulation.

The "good patient" phenomenon frequently emerges in therapeutic relationships with quiet BPD clients. These individuals arrive punctually, complete homework assignments diligently, and rarely challenge therapeutic boundaries or interventions. However, this compliance often masks intense internal struggles and may prevent authentic therapeutic engagement. Clinicians must look beyond surface-level cooperation to identify underlying emotional patterns and treatment needs.

Professional competence in treating quiet BPD requires ongoing education, consultation, and self-reflection. The subtle nature of symptoms, combined with clients' sophisticated masking abilities, can challenge even experienced clinicians' diagnostic accuracy and treatment planning skills. Understanding these unique presentations protects both clients and clinicians from therapeutic frustration and treatment failures.

Assessment strategies for hidden presentations

Traditional BPD assessment tools often fail to capture quiet BPD symptoms because they focus on externalized behaviors rather than internal experiences. Clients with quiet BPD typically score lower on standard measures while experiencing significant distress that doesn't translate into observable symptoms. This assessment gap requires modified approaches that identify internalized emotional dysregulation and self-directed destructive patterns.

Clinical interviewing techniques must probe beneath surface presentations. Standard mental health interviews may reveal minimal pathology when clients have mastered emotional concealment. Effective assessment requires specific questioning about internal experiences, self-criticism patterns, and subtle behavioral indicators that clients might not spontaneously report.

Dr. Rebecca Thompson, a clinician specializing in personality disorders, developed a modified assessment approach after repeatedly missing quiet BPD diagnoses during intake evaluations. She noticed that clients who initially presented with anxiety or depression often revealed more complex emotional patterns during deeper exploration of their internal experiences and relationship history.

Her assessment now includes specific questions about perfectionism, self-criticism, emotional numbness, and identity confusion. She asks about clients' internal dialogue, their comfort with making mistakes, and their experience of emotions in private versus public settings. This approach has significantly improved her diagnostic accuracy for quiet BPD presentations.

Observe discrepancies between reported and observed distress levels. Clients with quiet BPD often minimize their struggles while displaying subtle signs of significant emotional distress. Pay attention to clients who report being "fine" while demonstrating physical tension, emotional flatness, or exhaustion that seems disproportionate to their described experiences.

Sarah, a 32-year-old marketing executive, consistently reported that her life was "going well" during intake sessions. However, she appeared exhausted, spoke in a monotone voice, and described her daily routine in mechanistic terms that suggested emotional disconnection from her experiences. Further exploration revealed intense perfectionism, chronic emptiness, and identity confusion that she had never previously disclosed to a mental health professional.

Assess for subtle self-harm behaviors that don't involve obvious physical injury. Quiet BPD clients often engage in self-punitive behaviors that fly under the radar of standard self-harm assessments. These might include extreme exercise regimens, deliberate sleep deprivation, restrictive eating patterns, or engaging in situations that predictably cause emotional pain.

The assessment should explore how clients respond to mistakes, disappointments, or perceived failures. Do they engage in harsh self-criticism, punitive behaviors, or emotional self-attack that serves similar functions to more obvious forms of self-harm? Understanding these patterns is crucial for accurate diagnosis and treatment planning.

Evaluate emotional regulation strategies and their effectiveness. Clients with quiet BPD often develop sophisticated emotional regulation techniques that appear healthy on the surface but serve to suppress rather than process emotional experiences. They might rely heavily on intellectualization, compartmentalization, or extreme busyness to avoid emotional awareness.

Michael's assessment revealed that he used constant work engagement to avoid experiencing emotions. He worked 70-80 hours per week, not due to external demands, but because stopping work triggered overwhelming anxiety and emptiness. This pattern had allowed him to maintain professional success while preventing him from developing healthy emotional processing skills.

Explore identity and relationship patterns over time. Quiet BPD clients often struggle with identity confusion and relationship difficulties that become apparent only through detailed exploration of their history. They might describe feeling like they're "wearing masks" in different relationships or struggling to maintain authentic connections with others.

Assessment should explore clients' sense of self across different contexts, their comfort with intimacy and vulnerability, and their patterns in romantic relationships. Many quiet BPD clients have histories of brief, intense relationships that end when their emotional needs become too overwhelming to manage internally.

Countertransference with the "good patient"

Working with quiet BPD clients can trigger unique countertransference reactions that differ significantly from those experienced with traditional BPD presentations. The absence of obvious crisis behaviors, boundary violations, or dramatic presentations can lead clinicians to underestimate their clients' distress levels or treatment needs. Understanding and managing these reactions is essential for effective treatment.

The minimization trap affects both clients and clinicians. Quiet BPD clients' tendency to minimize their struggles can influence clinicians to similarly underestimate the severity of their symptoms. When clients consistently report that things are "fine" and don't present with crisis behaviors, clinicians might assume treatment is progressing well despite limited actual change in underlying patterns.

Dr. James Rodriguez experienced this dynamic with Elena, a client who attended sessions regularly, completed assignments, and reported gradual improvement in her anxiety symptoms. However, after six months of treatment, Elena's core emotional patterns remained unchanged. She continued to experience intense self-criticism, identity confusion, and relationship difficulties that she had learned to manage rather than resolve.

Dr. Rodriguez recognized that his satisfaction with Elena's compliance had prevented him from pushing deeper into her emotional experiences. He had unconsciously colluded with her avoidance patterns by accepting surface-level reports of progress without exploring underlying emotional dynamics.

Overprotectiveness can develop toward clients who seem fragile despite their competence. Quiet BPD clients often present as simultaneously competent and vulnerable, triggering clinicians' protective instincts. This can lead to avoiding challenging interventions, allowing clients to set the treatment pace entirely, or failing to address resistant behaviors that maintain their symptoms.

The challenge lies in recognizing clients' genuine vulnerability while maintaining therapeutic boundaries and challenging their avoidance patterns. Quiet BPD clients need clinicians who can see through their competent presentations to address underlying emotional needs without becoming overly protective or enabling their avoidance.

Boredom or therapeutic stuckness may indicate avoided emotional territory. Sessions with quiet BPD clients can feel superficial or repetitive, with clients reporting similar concerns week after week without apparent progress. This dynamic often indicates that both client and clinician are avoiding emotionally charged material that feels too dangerous to explore.

When treatment feels stuck, examine what emotional territories remain unexplored. Are there relationship patterns, family dynamics, or internal experiences that the client consistently steers away from? Is the therapeutic relationship itself being used to maintain emotional distance rather than promote genuine connection?

Admiration for clients' strength and competence can prevent recognition of their struggles. Quiet BPD clients often generate genuine admiration from clinicians who are impressed by their achievements, resilience, and apparent emotional regulation. While these qualities are real and admirable, focusing exclusively on strengths can prevent recognition of underlying vulnerabilities and treatment needs.

Dr. Lisa Chen found herself consistently impressed by David's professional accomplishments, thoughtful insights, and emotional maturity. However, this admiration prevented her from recognizing his profound loneliness, identity confusion, and fear of abandonment. Only when David experienced a major life transition did his underlying vulnerabilities become apparent, revealing the depth of his unaddressed emotional struggles.

Recognize the pull toward cognitive rather than emotional interventions. Quiet BPD clients' intellectual strengths and emotional avoidance can lead clinicians toward primarily cognitive treatment approaches that feel safer and more comfortable for both parties. While cognitive interventions have value, exclusive reliance on them may reinforce clients' existing patterns of emotional avoidance.

Effective treatment requires balancing cognitive understanding with emotional processing and experiential interventions that help clients access and tolerate previously avoided emotional experiences.

Treatment planning for overcontrolled clients

Quiet BPD clients typically present with overcontrolled rather than undercontrolled emotional patterns, requiring treatment approaches that differ significantly from traditional BPD interventions. Standard DBT protocols, which focus heavily on distress tolerance and emotional regulation skills, may need modification for clients whose primary challenge involves accessing and expressing emotions rather than managing emotional intensity.

Prioritize emotional awareness and expression over emotional regulation. Many quiet BPD clients have become experts at emotional suppression but struggle with emotional awareness and appropriate expression. Treatment planning should emphasize helping clients identify, tolerate, and express emotions that they have learned to suppress or avoid.

This might involve mindfulness practices focused on internal awareness, expressive therapies that facilitate emotional release, or behavioral experiments that gradually increase clients' comfort with emotional vulnerability. The goal is expanding emotional range rather than restricting it.

Address perfectionism as a core treatment target. Perfectionism often serves as both a coping mechanism and a maintaining factor for quiet BPD symptoms. Clients use perfectionist standards to avoid criticism and maintain control, but these same standards prevent them from taking emotional risks necessary for authentic relationships and personal growth.

Treatment should include specific interventions targeting perfectionist beliefs and behaviors. This might involve behavioral experiments with imperfection, cognitive restructuring of perfectionist standards, and gradual exposure to situations that trigger perfectionist anxiety.

Lisa's treatment plan specifically addressed her perfectionism through a series of planned "mistakes" and imperfections in low-stakes situations. She practiced submitting work assignments with minor errors, arriving slightly late to social events, and expressing opinions without extensive research or preparation. These exercises helped her develop tolerance for imperfection and reduced the emotional energy she expended maintaining perfect appearances.

Create treatment goals that balance symptom reduction with authentic self-expression. Quiet BPD clients often have difficulty identifying personal wants, needs, and preferences because they've focused extensively on meeting others' expectations and maintaining external success. Treatment planning should include goals related to identity development and authentic self-expression.

This might involve exploring personal values, preferences, and goals that exist independently of external validation. Clients need support in developing internal reference points for decision-making rather than relying exclusively on external feedback and approval.

Plan for gradual increase in interpersonal risk-taking. Quiet BPD clients typically maintain safe, surface-level relationships that protect them from rejection but prevent authentic connection. Treatment should include graduated exposure to interpersonal vulnerability and emotional intimacy.

Start with low-risk situations such as expressing minor preferences or disagreements, then gradually progress toward more significant emotional risks such as sharing personal struggles or setting boundaries in important relationships. The pace should be collaborative, with clients actively involved in determining their readiness for each level of interpersonal challenge.

Integrate individual and group treatment modalities. Quiet BPD clients often benefit from combination treatment approaches that provide both individual space for deep emotional work and group opportunities for interpersonal skill development. Group settings can be particularly valuable for clients who struggle with authentic self-expression and interpersonal connection.

However, group selection requires careful consideration. Traditional BPD process groups may feel overwhelming for clients who are just beginning to access their emotional experiences. Consider groups focused on specific skills such as assertiveness, interpersonal effectiveness, or emotional awareness rather than intensive process-oriented groups.

Supervision and consultation needs

Treating quiet BPD requires ongoing professional support and consultation due to the subtle nature of symptoms and the unique countertransference dynamics these clients can trigger. Even experienced clinicians benefit from external perspectives when working with clients whose presentations can be deceptively straightforward while involving complex underlying dynamics.

Seek consultation for diagnostic clarity and treatment planning. The subtle nature of quiet BPD symptoms can create diagnostic uncertainty, particularly when clients present with comorbid conditions such as anxiety, depression, or eating disorders. Regular consultation helps clinicians distinguish between primary and secondary diagnoses and develop treatment plans that address core emotional patterns rather than surface symptoms.

Dr. Patricia Williams regularly consulted with colleagues about her quiet BPD cases because she found their presentations could be misleadingly simple. Clients who initially appeared to have straightforward anxiety or depression often revealed more complex emotional patterns that required significant treatment plan modifications. Consultation helped her recognize these patterns earlier and develop more effective interventions.

Use supervision to identify countertransference patterns. The "good patient" phenomenon and other unique countertransference reactions can be difficult to recognize without external feedback. Regular supervision provides opportunities to explore clinicians' emotional reactions, identify potential blind spots, and develop strategies for managing challenging therapeutic dynamics.

Supervision should specifically address clinicians' comfort with challenging compliant clients, their ability to recognize minimization and avoidance, and their skills in balancing support with appropriate therapeutic pressure.

Develop case formulations collaboratively. Quiet BPD presentations can benefit from multiple clinical perspectives due to their complexity and subtlety. Team case formulation meetings or consultation groups can provide valuable insights into clients' underlying dynamics and treatment needs that individual clinicians might miss.

These collaborative formulations should integrate multiple theoretical perspectives and consider how clients' strengths and competencies might also serve as defenses against emotional intimacy and authentic self-expression.

Access specialized training in overcontrolled presentations. Traditional BPD training often focuses on managing undercontrolled behaviors and dramatic presentations. Clinicians working with quiet BPD benefit from specialized training in approaches such as Radically Open DBT, which specifically addresses overcontrolled emotional patterns.

This training should cover assessment techniques for identifying subtle symptoms, intervention strategies for promoting emotional expression and interpersonal risk-taking, and approaches for managing the unique therapeutic challenges these clients present.

Establish ongoing education about personality disorder research.
The understanding of quiet BPD and overcontrolled presentations
continues to evolve, with new research regularly emerging about
assessment, treatment, and long-term outcomes. Clinicians should
maintain current knowledge through professional literature, continuing
education, and specialized training opportunities.

Clinical Resources: Assessment tools and treatment protocols

Several specialized assessment tools and treatment protocols have
been developed specifically for identifying and treating overcontrolled
presentations and quiet BPD symptoms. These resources can
significantly improve diagnostic accuracy and treatment effectiveness
for clients whose symptoms don't align with traditional BPD
presentations.

The Overcontrol Scale (OCS) measures emotional overcontrol
patterns that characterize quiet BPD presentations. This assessment
tool evaluates rigid and rule-governed behavior, low emotional
expression, and social isolation patterns that traditional BPD measures
might miss. The OCS helps clinicians identify clients who would
benefit from interventions focused on increasing emotional expression
and interpersonal connection rather than emotional regulation.

The Inventory of Interpersonal Problems-64 provides detailed
assessment of interpersonal difficulties that quiet BPD clients
commonly experience. This tool identifies specific patterns such as
difficulty being assertive, problems with intimacy, and tendencies
toward social inhibition that inform treatment planning and
intervention selection.

Radically Open Dialectical Behavior Therapy (RO-DBT)
represents a specialized treatment protocol developed specifically for
overcontrolled presentations. Unlike traditional DBT, which focuses
on emotional regulation and distress tolerance, RO-DBT emphasizes
increasing emotional expression, interpersonal connection, and
behavioral flexibility.

192

The protocol includes specific skills modules for enhancing emotional awareness, promoting authentic self-expression, and developing healthy interpersonal connections. Treatment incorporates mindfulness practices designed to increase emotional sensitivity rather than emotional regulation.

The Schema Therapy model provides another framework for understanding and treating quiet BPD presentations. This approach identifies specific schema patterns such as defectiveness/shame, emotional inhibition, and unrelenting standards that commonly characterize quiet BPD clients. Schema Therapy techniques can be particularly effective for addressing core identity issues and relationship patterns.

Mentalization-Based Treatment (MBT) focuses on developing clients' capacity to understand their own and others' mental states. This approach can be particularly valuable for quiet BPD clients who struggle with emotional awareness and interpersonal connection. MBT techniques help clients develop more sophisticated understanding of emotional experiences and improve their capacity for authentic relationships.

Professional competence in treating quiet BPD requires specialized knowledge, modified assessment strategies, and adapted treatment approaches that differ significantly from traditional BPD interventions. The subtlety of symptoms and clients' sophisticated masking abilities challenge clinicians to develop enhanced sensitivity to hidden emotional patterns while maintaining therapeutic boundaries and effectiveness.

The "good patient" phenomenon represents both a gift and a challenge in therapeutic relationships. While these clients' cooperation and insight facilitate certain aspects of treatment, their compliance can mask avoidance patterns that maintain their symptoms. Clinicians must balance appreciation for clients' strengths with recognition of their underlying vulnerabilities and treatment needs.

193

Ongoing professional development, consultation, and supervision are essential components of effective quiet BPD treatment. The complexity and subtlety of these presentations require external perspectives and specialized training to maintain diagnostic accuracy and treatment effectiveness. Investment in these professional supports ultimately benefits both clinicians and the clients they serve.

Key Takeaways for Clinical Practice:

- Develop assessment strategies that probe beneath surface presentations to identify internalized emotional dysregulation patterns
- Recognize and manage unique countertransference reactions triggered by compliant, high-functioning clients who minimize their distress
- Adapt treatment planning to address overcontrolled rather than undercontrolled emotional patterns, emphasizing expression over regulation
- Utilize specialized assessment tools and treatment protocols designed specifically for overcontrolled presentations
- Maintain ongoing consultation and supervision to navigate the subtle dynamics and complex presentations these clients bring
- Invest in specialized training and continuing education to stay current with evolving understanding of quiet BPD treatment approaches

Chapter 18: Building communities of understanding

The journey of understanding and healing from quiet BPD often feels profoundly isolating. Unlike more visible mental health conditions, quiet BPD symptoms remain hidden beneath successful external presentations, making it difficult for individuals to recognize their experiences in others or find communities of people who truly understand their struggles. Building authentic connections requires courage to move beyond surface-level interactions and seek spaces where emotional honesty and vulnerability are welcomed rather than feared.

Traditional mental health support systems often fail to address the unique needs of people with quiet BPD. Support groups designed for general anxiety or depression may not resonate with individuals whose symptoms involve complex identity issues, perfectionism, and fear of abandonment masked by high achievement and emotional control. Generic wellness advice rarely addresses the sophisticated emotional regulation strategies that both protect and imprison people with quiet BPD.

Creating meaningful communities requires understanding the specific barriers that prevent people with quiet BPD from engaging authentically with others. Their fear of being seen as flawed or needy, combined with their expertise at maintaining perfect appearances, can prevent them from accessing the very connections that promote healing. Effective community building must address these barriers while providing safe spaces for gradual emotional vulnerability and authentic self-expression.

Support groups: Finding your people

Support groups specifically designed for quiet BPD or overcontrolled presentations offer unique benefits that general mental health support cannot provide. These specialized groups understand the internal experience of maintaining perfect external appearances while struggling with intense emotional pain, identity confusion, and relationship difficulties that remain largely invisible to others.

In-person support groups create opportunities for authentic connection. Meeting face-to-face with others who share similar struggles can be powerfully validating for people who have spent years believing they were uniquely flawed or abnormal. Seeing others who appear successful and competent while sharing similar internal experiences helps normalize their struggles and reduces shame about their hidden difficulties.

The Quiet BPD Support Circle in Seattle began when therapist Dr. Amanda Foster noticed that several of her clients expressed frustration about not fitting into traditional BPD support groups. The clients felt their experiences were minimized or misunderstood by group members whose symptoms were more externally visible. Dr. Foster partnered with a local mental health center to create a specialized group focused specifically on internalizing presentations.

The group meets weekly for 90 minutes and includes 8-12 participants who rotate through different phases of involvement based on their treatment needs and life circumstances. Members appreciate the group's focus on perfectionism, emotional suppression, and the unique challenges of maintaining professional success while managing internal emotional chaos.

Sarah, a group member for two years, credits the support circle with helping her understand that her struggles were real and valid even though they didn't match traditional mental illness presentations. "For the first time, I met people who understood what it felt like to be dying inside while everyone told you how successful and together you seemed," she explains.

Peer-led support groups offer different benefits than professionally facilitated groups. While professional facilitation provides structure and clinical expertise, peer-led groups often create more egalitarian environments where members can explore their experiences without feeling evaluated or diagnosed. These groups can be particularly valuable for people with quiet BPD who are sensitive to power dynamics and evaluation by authority figures.

The Online Quiet Warriors support group started as an informal Facebook group and evolved into a structured peer-led organization with regional chapters across North America. Members take turns facilitating meetings, sharing resources, and providing support during crisis periods. The group emphasizes mutual aid and shared leadership rather than traditional therapeutic models.

Members report that peer leadership feels less threatening than professional facilitation and allows for more spontaneous, authentic sharing. The absence of clinical oversight also permits discussions about treatment frustrations, therapy relationships, and mental health system navigation that might feel inappropriate in professionally led groups.

Support groups must balance structure with flexibility. People with quiet BPD often struggle with rigid thinking and benefit from environments that model flexibility while maintaining enough structure to feel safe. Effective groups establish clear guidelines about confidentiality, respect, and participation while allowing for organic discussion and emotional expression.

The Minneapolis Quiet BPD Circle uses a flexible format that includes brief check-ins, themed discussions, and open sharing time. Topics rotate based on member interests and current needs, covering subjects such as workplace stress management, relationship boundaries, family dynamics, and treatment experiences. The structure provides predictability while allowing for spontaneous exploration of emerging issues.

Groups should address the unique challenges of high-functioning presentations. Unlike traditional BPD support groups that might focus on crisis management and basic life skills, quiet BPD groups need to address the specific challenges of maintaining external success while managing internal emotional struggles. This includes workplace stress, perfectionism in parenting, relationship maintenance, and identity development in the context of external achievement.

Discussions often focus on topics such as impostor syndrome, overcommitment patterns, difficulty saying no, and the exhaustion of maintaining perfect appearances. Members explore strategies for gradual vulnerability, authentic self-expression, and sustainable life balance that don't require abandoning their competencies and achievements.

Online communities: Benefits and boundaries

Digital platforms offer unique advantages for quiet BPD support, particularly for individuals who struggle with in-person vulnerability or have limited access to specialized local resources. However, online communities also present specific risks that require careful navigation to maintain their therapeutic value while avoiding potential harm.

Online anonymity can facilitate initial vulnerability. Many people with quiet BPD find it easier to share authentically in digital environments where they can control their identity presentation and maintain privacy. Screen names and avatars allow for emotional honesty without the exposure fears that prevent in-person sharing.

The Reddit community r/QuietBPD has grown to over 45,000 members who share experiences, resources, and support through posts and comments. Members often begin participation by reading others' experiences before gradually sharing their own struggles. The anonymity allows people to explore difficult topics such as self-harm, relationship patterns, and family dysfunction without fear of professional or personal consequences.

Marcus discovered the community during a particularly difficult period when he was struggling with work stress and relationship issues but couldn't bring himself to seek in-person support. Reading posts from others who described experiences similar to his own helped him recognize patterns he had never identified as symptoms of a diagnosable condition. The community provided education and validation that ultimately led him to seek professional treatment.

Virtual support groups can supplement in-person treatment. Video-based support groups offer some benefits of face-to-face interaction while maintaining the accessibility of digital platforms. These groups can be particularly valuable for people in rural areas, those with mobility limitations, or individuals whose work schedules make regular in-person attendance difficult.

The Zoom-based Quiet BPD Weekly Circle serves members across multiple time zones with rotating meeting times to accommodate different schedules. The group uses breakout rooms for smaller discussion groups and incorporates guided meditation and mindfulness exercises that participants can practice at home. Members report that seeing others' faces and hearing their voices creates more connection than text-based communities while remaining more accessible than in-person groups.

Online communities require active moderation to maintain therapeutic value. Without proper oversight, online mental health communities can devolve into crisis escalation, toxic positivity, or harmful advice sharing. Effective quiet BPD online communities establish clear guidelines about appropriate content, crisis response protocols, and consequences for harmful behavior.

The Facebook group "Quiet BPD Support and Understanding" employs a team of volunteer moderators who have experience with quiet BPD and training in online community management. The group maintains strict rules about no diagnosis giving, no medical advice, and no detailed descriptions of self-harm methods. Moderators monitor posts for concerning content and have protocols for referring members to professional crisis resources when needed.

Digital boundaries protect both individuals and communities. Online participation can become compulsive for people with quiet BPD who struggle with emotional regulation and seek constant validation. Communities should encourage healthy boundaries around screen time, emotional support seeking, and crisis communication.

Effective online communities establish guidelines about appropriate support requests, time limits for crisis discussions, and expectations for reciprocal rather than one-sided support relationships. Members learn to recognize when online interaction becomes avoidance of in-person relationships or professional treatment rather than a supplement to comprehensive care.

Information sharing requires careful curation. Online communities often share resources about treatment options, mental health professionals, and coping strategies. However, the decentralized nature of digital platforms makes quality control challenging. Communities must balance open information sharing with responsible curation to prevent misinformation or harmful advice.

The website QuietBPDResources.org maintains a curated database of treatment providers, assessment tools, and educational materials specifically focused on quiet BPD and overcontrolled presentations. The site's editorial board includes mental health professionals and community members who review submissions for accuracy and appropriateness before publication. This approach provides comprehensive resources while maintaining quality standards.

Peer support models that work

Effective peer support for quiet BPD requires models that address the specific challenges these individuals face in forming authentic connections while leveraging their strengths and capabilities. Traditional peer support approaches may need modification to accommodate the unique presentation patterns and needs of people with quiet BPD.

Mentorship programs pair individuals at different stages of recovery. People with quiet BPD often benefit from seeing examples of others who have successfully navigated similar struggles while maintaining their professional competence and personal achievements.

Mentorship relationships provide hope, practical guidance, and modeling of healthy emotional expression within the context of continued success.

The Quiet Strength Mentorship Program matches individuals newly diagnosed with quiet BPD with mentors who have at least two years of treatment experience and demonstrated progress in emotional awareness and interpersonal connections. Mentors receive training in boundary setting, crisis response, and appropriate support provision to ensure relationships remain helpful rather than becoming codependent.

Jennifer, a mentor in the program, meets monthly with her mentee Lisa to discuss treatment progress, workplace challenges, and relationship development. Jennifer shares her own recovery journey while avoiding giving advice or becoming responsible for Lisa's treatment outcomes. The relationship provides Lisa with hope that recovery is possible while maintaining professional success and personal competence.

Buddy systems provide ongoing support between formal meetings. People with quiet BPD often struggle during the periods between therapy appointments or support group meetings when they feel isolated with their internal struggles. Buddy relationships provide regular contact and support without the intensity or commitment of formal mentorship relationships.

The Seattle Quiet BPD Support Circle pairs members who volunteer for buddy relationships based on similar life circumstances, interests, or treatment goals. Buddies commit to weekly check-in calls and are available for brief support during difficult periods. The relationships are reciprocal, with both partners providing and receiving support rather than one person serving as helper and the other as helped.

Boundaries are clearly established to prevent buddy relationships from becoming therapeutic or codependent. Partners focus on emotional support, resource sharing, and social connection rather than problem-solving or crisis intervention, which remain the responsibility of professional treatment providers.

Skill-sharing workshops leverage members' professional competencies. Many people with quiet BPD possess significant professional skills and expertise that can benefit others in the community. Skill-sharing workshops allow members to contribute their strengths while building connections and reducing the shame often associated with receiving help.

The Phoenix Quiet BPD Community organizes monthly workshops where members teach skills related to their professional expertise while connecting those skills to mental health and recovery topics. Recent workshops have included "Mindful Communication for Lawyers," "Financial Planning for Emotional Stability," "Project Management for Life Balance," and "Creative Expression for Engineers."

These workshops serve multiple functions: they provide valuable skills to participants, allow presenters to contribute meaningfully to the community, and demonstrate that people with quiet BPD can maintain professional competence while addressing their emotional needs. The format reduces stigma and promotes a sense of mutual contribution rather than one-way help receiving.

Recovery story sharing provides hope and practical guidance. People with quiet BPD often struggle to envision what recovery looks like given their high-functioning presentations. Recovery stories from others with similar experiences provide concrete examples of how treatment and personal growth can occur without requiring dramatic life changes or abandoning professional success.

The online platform "Quiet Voices: Recovery Stories" features written and video testimonials from people at various stages of recovery from quiet BPD. Stories include specific details about treatment approaches, relationship changes, career impacts, and ongoing challenges to provide realistic rather than idealized recovery portrayals.

Contributors share their real names and photos to demonstrate that recovery from quiet BPD doesn't require hiding or shame about mental health treatment. Stories emphasize gradual progress, ongoing challenges, and the integration of treatment with continued professional and personal success.

Advocacy and awareness building

Raising awareness about quiet BPD serves multiple purposes: it helps undiagnosed individuals recognize their symptoms and seek appropriate treatment, educates mental health professionals about these presentations, and reduces stigma about high-functioning mental illness. However, advocacy efforts must be carefully planned to avoid sensationalizing or misrepresenting the condition.

Educational campaigns target multiple audiences with tailored messaging. Effective quiet BPD awareness efforts recognize that different groups need different types of information presented in formats that resonate with their specific concerns and knowledge levels. Messages for potential patients differ significantly from those designed for mental health professionals or family members.

The "Hidden Struggles" awareness campaign developed by the Quiet BPD Foundation creates separate educational materials for individuals who might have quiet BPD, their family members, and mental health professionals. Materials for potential patients focus on symptom recognition and treatment options, family materials emphasize support strategies and boundary setting, and professional materials provide assessment tools and treatment recommendations.

Campaign materials avoid dramatic or sensationalized presentations that might reinforce stigma or create misconceptions about the condition. Instead, they focus on accurate information, hope for recovery, and the importance of professional assessment and treatment.

Professional education initiatives improve diagnostic accuracy and treatment outcomes. Many mental health professionals have limited training in recognizing and treating quiet BPD presentations. Educational initiatives for clinicians can significantly improve access to appropriate care for people with these symptoms.

203

The annual Quiet BPD Clinical Conference brings together researchers, clinicians, and individuals with lived experience to share current knowledge about assessment, treatment, and recovery. The conference features presentations on diagnostic criteria, evidence-based treatments, and emerging research while maintaining focus on practical clinical applications.

Conference participants report increased confidence in identifying quiet BPD presentations and greater awareness of appropriate treatment modifications for overcontrolled clients. Follow-up surveys indicate that attendees modify their assessment practices and treatment approaches based on conference learning.

Stigma reduction efforts emphasize competence alongside struggle. Traditional mental health stigma reduction campaigns often focus on dramatic recovery stories or emphasize that people with mental illness are "just like everyone else." For quiet BPD, effective anti-stigma efforts must address the unique challenges of high-functioning presentations while avoiding minimization of genuine struggles.

The "Success and Struggle" media campaign features stories of professionals, parents, students, and community leaders who have quiet BPD and have integrated treatment into their lives while maintaining their competence and achievements. Stories emphasize both the reality of internal struggles and the possibility of successful treatment without requiring life disruption.

Campaign messages challenge assumptions that successful, competent people cannot have serious mental health needs while also demonstrating that mental health treatment can enhance rather than threaten professional and personal success.

Resource Directory: Organizations and support networks

Building comprehensive resource networks for quiet BPD requires coordination between professional organizations, advocacy groups, treatment providers, and peer support communities. Effective resource directories provide multiple types of support while maintaining quality standards and accessibility.

Treatment provider directories specialize in quiet BPD expertise. General mental health provider directories often don't identify clinicians with specific expertise in quiet BPD or overcontrolled presentations. Specialized directories help individuals find appropriate treatment while helping qualified clinicians connect with clients who need their expertise.

The Quiet BPD Treatment Network maintains a searchable database of mental health professionals who have specialized training in treating overcontrolled presentations. Providers must meet specific qualification criteria including specialized training, supervision experience, and ongoing education in quiet BPD treatment approaches.

The directory includes information about treatment modalities offered, insurance acceptance, availability for new clients, and geographic service areas. Client reviews and outcome data help individuals make informed choices about treatment providers while maintaining appropriate professional boundaries.

Crisis resource networks address unique quiet BPD needs. Traditional crisis hotlines may not be prepared to address the specific needs of people with quiet BPD who are experiencing emotional crises while maintaining external functioning. Specialized crisis resources understand these presentations and can provide appropriate support.

The Quiet Crisis Support Network trains volunteers specifically in supporting people with overcontrolled presentations who are experiencing emotional crises. Volunteers understand that callers might appear highly functional while experiencing genuine emotional emergencies and are trained to provide validation and support without minimizing their struggles.

The network maintains relationships with mental health professionals who specialize in quiet BPD to facilitate appropriate referrals and follow-up care. Crisis supporters focus on immediate safety and connection to ongoing resources rather than attempting to provide ongoing therapeutic support.

Educational resource libraries curate high-quality information. The abundance of online mental health information makes it difficult for individuals to identify accurate, helpful resources specific to quiet BPD. Curated libraries provide quality-controlled access to educational materials, self-help resources, and treatment information.

The Quiet BPD Resource Library partners with mental health professionals, researchers, and advocacy organizations to maintain a comprehensive collection of books, articles, videos, and online resources specifically focused on quiet BPD and overcontrolled presentations. Materials are reviewed for accuracy and appropriateness before inclusion.

The library includes sections for individuals with quiet BPD, family members, mental health professionals, and researchers. Resources are organized by topic and difficulty level to help users find materials appropriate to their needs and knowledge levels.

Building communities of understanding for quiet BPD requires intentional effort to create spaces where authenticity is safe and valued. These communities serve as bridges between isolation and connection, providing opportunities for people to share their hidden struggles while maintaining their competencies and achievements.

Effective community building recognizes that people with quiet BPD need specialized approaches that address their unique presentation patterns and challenges. Generic mental health support often fails to resonate with their experiences, while communities designed specifically for their needs can provide profound validation and practical assistance.

The development of strong support networks benefits not only individuals with quiet BPD but also their families, treatment providers, and broader communities. When people with quiet BPD have access to understanding and support, they can contribute more authentically to their relationships and professional environments while managing their symptoms more effectively.

Key Takeaways for Community Building:

- Seek specialized support groups that understand the unique challenges of maintaining external success while managing internal struggles
- Use online communities as supplements to rather than replacements for in-person connections and professional treatment
- Participate in peer support models that leverage your strengths while providing opportunities for authentic connection and mutual assistance
- Support advocacy efforts that accurately represent quiet BPD while reducing stigma and improving access to appropriate care
- Utilize curated resource directories to find qualified treatment providers and high-quality educational materials specific to your needs
- Contribute to community building efforts by sharing your experiences and expertise in ways that feel comfortable and sustainable

Chapter 19: Recovery journeys: Five stories of quiet courage

Recovery from quiet BPD rarely follows a linear path or dramatic transformation narrative. Instead, it unfolds through gradual shifts in self-awareness, incremental changes in relationship patterns, and slowly developing comfort with emotional authenticity. The individuals whose stories follow represent diverse backgrounds, ages, and life circumstances, yet they share common themes of courage, persistence, and the willingness to challenge deeply ingrained patterns of emotional concealment.

These stories illustrate that recovery doesn't require abandoning competence or success. Rather, it involves integrating emotional awareness and authentic self-expression with existing strengths and capabilities. Each person found their own path through the maze of perfectionism, people-pleasing, and emotional suppression that characterizes quiet BPD, discovering that healing could coexist with professional achievement and personal responsibility.

The journeys described here span multiple years and include setbacks, breakthroughs, and periods of plateau that characterize authentic recovery processes. They demonstrate that quiet BPD recovery is possible while maintaining the achievements and relationships that matter most to individuals with this condition.

Holly's four-year transformation

Holly's story begins with what appeared to be a perfect life falling apart in slow motion. At 29, she held a senior marketing position at a prestigious firm, lived in a downtown apartment she had decorated with magazine-worthy precision, and maintained an Instagram presence that generated envious comments from friends and strangers alike. Behind this carefully curated exterior, Holly was drowning in anxiety, perfectionism, and a bone-deep loneliness that no amount of external validation could touch.

The first crack in Holly's facade appeared during a routine performance review when her supervisor mentioned that she seemed "wound too tight" and suggested she take some vacation time. The comment triggered weeks of obsessive analysis about her workplace behavior and desperate attempts to appear more relaxed while maintaining her perfectionist work standards. She began experiencing panic attacks that she attributed to coffee consumption and worked even harder to compensate for what she perceived as declining performance.

Holly's breaking point came during her annual family Christmas gathering when her younger sister casually mentioned feeling concerned about Holly's obvious exhaustion and withdrawal from family interactions. The observation, delivered with love and genuine care, felt like a devastating critique of Holly's ability to maintain her perfect image even within her own family.

"I had spent so much energy making sure everyone saw me as successful and together that I had no idea who I actually was underneath all that performance," Holly reflects. "My sister's comment made me realize that even my closest relationships were based on a version of me that wasn't real."

Holly's initial therapy attempts focused on anxiety management and work-life balance, approaches that provided temporary relief but didn't address her underlying emotional patterns. She learned breathing techniques and time management strategies while continuing to experience the emptiness and identity confusion that drove her perfectionist behaviors.

The breakthrough came when Holly began working with a therapist trained in treating quiet BPD presentations. For the first time, she encountered a professional who recognized her high functioning as a sophisticated defense mechanism rather than evidence that her struggles weren't serious. The therapist helped Holly understand that her perfectionism, people-pleasing, and emotional suppression were symptoms of a treatable condition rather than character flaws or personal weaknesses.

Holly's second year of recovery involved the difficult work of learning to tolerate imperfection in small, manageable doses. She practiced submitting work projects without excessive revision, expressing minor disagreements in meetings, and declining social invitations when she felt genuinely tired rather than forcing herself to maintain constant availability.

These changes felt terrifying initially. Holly worried that showing any imperfection would result in professional consequences, relationship loss, or confirmation of her deepest fears about being fundamentally flawed. Instead, she discovered that most people responded positively to her increased authenticity and that her work quality actually improved when she stopped obsessing over minor details.

The most challenging aspect of Holly's recovery involved learning to identify and express her genuine emotions and preferences. Having spent years suppressing her internal experiences in favor of external expectations, Holly initially had no idea what she actually wanted or felt in most situations. She had to learn to sit with uncertainty and gradually develop internal awareness that could guide her decision-making.

"I realized I had no idea what I actually liked or disliked because I had spent so long figuring out what I should like," Holly explains. "Learning to have preferences felt incredibly selfish at first, but it was actually the beginning of becoming a real person instead of a performance."

Holly's relationship patterns underwent significant changes during her third year of recovery. She had historically maintained surface-level friendships based on shared activities or professional networking rather than emotional connection. Recovery required evaluating these relationships and gradually increasing vulnerability with people who demonstrated trustworthiness and genuine care.

Some relationships didn't survive Holly's increased authenticity. Friends who had appreciated her constant availability and problem-solving assistance became uncomfortable when she began setting boundaries and expressing her own needs. However, other relationships deepened significantly as Holly learned to share struggles, ask for support, and engage in reciprocal rather than one-sided caring.

Holly's family relationships required particularly careful navigation. Her parents had always praised her independence and success, inadvertently reinforcing her belief that love was contingent on perfect performance. Recovery involved helping her family understand that their well-intentioned praise for her strength had contributed to her reluctance to show vulnerability or ask for help.

Four years into her recovery journey, Holly describes her life as "messier but more real." She still maintains professional success and personal achievement, but these accomplishments no longer define her entire sense of worth. She has learned to tolerate mistakes, express disagreement, and prioritize her emotional wellbeing alongside external responsibilities.

Holly's current challenges involve maintaining her recovery gains during stressful periods and continuing to develop emotional intimacy in her romantic relationships. She recognizes that recovery is an ongoing process rather than a destination and has learned to view setbacks as information rather than failures.

"I used to think recovery would mean becoming a completely different person, but it actually meant becoming more of who I already was underneath all the fear and performance," Holly reflects. "I'm still ambitious and capable, but now those qualities serve me rather than consuming me."

M.K.'s lotus flower renewal

M.K.'s journey toward understanding and healing from quiet BPD began in the aftermath of a divorce that shattered her carefully constructed identity as the perfect wife, mother, and community member. At 42, she had spent nearly two decades building a life that

211

appeared enviably successful from the outside while feeling increasingly empty and inauthentic on the inside.

The marriage had functioned smoothly for years based on M.K.'s willingness to adapt herself to her husband's needs and preferences while suppressing her own desires and opinions. She managed their social calendar, maintained their home, and coordinated their children's activities with efficiency that earned admiration from other parents. However, this external success came at the cost of her own identity and emotional wellbeing.

M.K.'s husband initiated the divorce after years of growing apart, citing their lack of genuine connection and his feeling that he "didn't really know who she was." The accusation felt devastating because M.K. realized it was accurate – she had no idea who she was beyond her roles as wife and mother. She had spent so long being what others needed that she had lost touch with her own authentic self.

"I had become a human chameleon," M.K. explains. "I was so good at reading what people wanted and becoming that person that I forgot I was supposed to have my own wants and needs too."

The divorce proceedings revealed the extent to which M.K. had abdicated responsibility for her own life. She had no clear preferences about living arrangements, financial decisions, or custody schedules because she had never developed the skill of knowing what she actually wanted. Her attorney grew frustrated with her inability to advocate for herself and suggested she seek counseling to clarify her goals and priorities.

M.K.'s initial therapy focused on practical decision-making skills and assertiveness training. While these approaches provided some benefit, they didn't address the underlying emotional patterns that had led to her self-abandonment. She learned to express preferences but felt guilty and selfish whenever she prioritized her own needs over others' wants.

The turning point came when M.K.'s therapist introduced the concept of quiet BPD and helped her understand that her people-pleasing and identity confusion were symptoms of a recognizable condition rather than personal failures. For the first time, M.K. had language to describe her internal experience and hope that change was possible.

M.K. chose the lotus flower as her recovery symbol after learning that these plants grow through mud and murky water to bloom on the surface. The metaphor resonated deeply with her experience of finding beauty and authenticity through the difficult process of examining her suppressed emotions and abandoned dreams.

The first year of M.K.'s recovery involved grieving the life she had thought she wanted while exploring who she might become. She had to confront the reality that many of her previous choices had been based on others' expectations rather than her own values and preferences. This process felt simultaneously liberating and terrifying as she contemplated building a life based on her authentic self.

M.K. began experimenting with small acts of self-expression that felt manageable. She redecorated her new apartment according to her own aesthetic preferences rather than design trends or others' opinions. She tried new hobbies and activities to discover what brought her genuine joy rather than what she thought she should enjoy.

The most challenging aspect of M.K.'s recovery involved learning to tolerate disapproval and conflict. Having spent decades avoiding disagreement by constantly accommodating others, she had to develop entirely new skills for handling situations where her needs conflicted with others' wants.

This learning process proved particularly difficult in her relationship with her teenage children, who had grown accustomed to their mother's constant availability and accommodation. When M.K. began setting boundaries and expressing her own needs, her children initially responded with confusion and resistance.

"They kept asking why I was being so selfish all of a sudden," M.K. recalls. "It took time for all of us to understand that taking care of myself actually made me a better mother because I wasn't resentful and exhausted all the time."

M.K.'s second year of recovery involved exploring career possibilities that aligned with her authentic interests rather than others' expectations. Having worked part-time in administrative roles to accommodate her family's needs, she had never seriously considered what type of work might fulfill her personally.

Through career counseling and volunteer experiences, M.K. discovered a passion for helping other women navigate life transitions. She began training as a divorce coach and eventually started her own practice focused on supporting women through major life changes.

The career transition required M.K. to challenge her beliefs about her capabilities and worthiness. Having spent years defining herself through others' achievements, she had to learn to value her own insights, skills, and contributions. Building a successful practice while maintaining her recovery required constant attention to balancing ambition with self-care.

Three years into her recovery, M.K. began dating again – a process that triggered many of her old patterns around identity adaptation and people-pleasing. She had to learn to maintain her authentic self in romantic relationships while remaining open to genuine connection and compromise.

"Dating in recovery meant learning to show up as myself from the beginning instead of trying to figure out what the other person wanted and becoming that," M.K. explains. "It was scary because it meant risking rejection for who I actually was, but it also meant any relationship that developed would be based on reality."

M.K.'s current relationship, which began four years into her recovery, represents the first romantic partnership where she has maintained her authentic identity while building genuine intimacy. Her partner knows about her quiet BPD diagnosis and recovery journey, and they have developed communication patterns that support both of their emotional wellbeing.

Five years after her divorce, M.K. describes her life as "unrecognizable in the best possible way." She maintains strong relationships with her children while modeling healthy boundaries and self-care. Her coaching practice thrives because she can offer authentic support based on her own recovery experience.

M.K.'s ongoing recovery challenges include managing perfectionist tendencies in her new career and continuing to develop emotional intimacy without losing herself in relationships. She remains committed to therapy and personal growth while enjoying the life she has built based on her authentic values and preferences.

"The lotus became my symbol because it reminded me that beautiful things can grow from difficult circumstances," M.K. reflects. "My divorce felt like the end of everything, but it was actually the beginning of my real life."

Rachel's advocacy awakening

Rachel's quiet BPD diagnosis came at age 35 during what appeared to be the peak of her success as a corporate attorney. She had recently made partner at a prestigious firm, owned a beautiful home, and maintained an active social life that included charity work and professional networking. However, beneath this impressive exterior, Rachel struggled with chronic anxiety, impostor syndrome, and a pervasive sense that she was living someone else's life.

The catalyst for seeking help came during a high-profile case when Rachel experienced what she later recognized as a panic attack during a crucial client meeting. She managed to complete the meeting professionally but spent the remainder of the day in her office bathroom, crying and struggling to breathe. The incident terrified her because it represented a crack in the perfect professional image she had worked years to maintain.

Rachel's initial attempts to address her symptoms focused on stress management and work-life balance strategies. She tried meditation apps, yoga classes, and time management techniques while continuing to work 70-hour weeks and maintain her extensive social and professional commitments. These approaches provided minimal relief because they didn't address the underlying emotional patterns driving her overcommitment and perfectionism.

The breakthrough came when Rachel began working with a therapist who specialized in treating high-functioning professionals with personality disorders. For the first time, Rachel encountered someone who understood that her professional success was both genuine achievement and sophisticated avoidance mechanism.

"I had always thought that being successful meant I couldn't have serious mental health problems," Rachel explains. "Learning about quiet BPD helped me understand that my perfectionism and people-pleasing weren't just personality quirks – they were symptoms of something that could be treated."

Rachel's early recovery involved learning to recognize and challenge her perfectionist thinking patterns. She had to confront the reality that her fear of making mistakes was preventing her from taking appropriate risks and growing professionally. Her terror of disappointing others was causing her to overcommit and underperform due to exhaustion.

The process of change felt particularly threatening because Rachel's identity was so tightly connected to her professional competence. She worried that addressing her emotional patterns would somehow diminish her capabilities or success. Instead, she discovered that increased self-awareness and emotional regulation actually enhanced her professional effectiveness.

Rachel's second year of recovery involved gradually increasing her comfort with vulnerability and authentic self-expression. She began sharing struggles with trusted colleagues rather than maintaining the image that everything came easily to her. She started declining committee assignments and social invitations that didn't align with her genuine interests or energy levels.

These changes initially felt selfish and scary. Rachel had built her professional reputation on being constantly available and willing to handle any assignment. Learning to set boundaries required developing new skills in communication and prioritization while managing her fear of disappointing others.

The most transformative aspect of Rachel's recovery involved recognizing how her quiet BPD symptoms affected not only her own wellbeing but also her ability to support others effectively. She began to understand that her constant self-sacrifice and emotional suppression were modeling unhealthy patterns for junior colleagues and contributing to toxic workplace dynamics.

This realization sparked Rachel's interest in advocacy and systemic change. She began researching workplace mental health issues and discovered that many high-performing professionals struggled with similar patterns of perfectionism, overcommitment, and emotional suppression without recognizing these as symptoms of treatable conditions.

Rachel's advocacy efforts began small, with informal mentoring relationships where she shared her recovery experience with junior colleagues who seemed to be struggling with similar patterns. She was surprised by how many people expressed relief at hearing their experiences validated and normalized rather than pathologized.

Encouraged by these positive responses, Rachel began speaking about mental health and perfectionism at professional development events. Her presentations focused on the intersection of high achievement and emotional wellbeing, challenging the assumption that professional success indicated overall wellness.

"I started realizing that my recovery could help other people avoid years of suffering if they could recognize these patterns earlier,"

217

Rachel explains. "It felt like a way to make something positive out of my own struggles."

Rachel's advocacy work expanded to include writing articles for professional publications about workplace mental health, particularly the unique challenges faced by high-achieving individuals with internalizing mental health conditions. Her articles resonated with readers who had never seen their experiences reflected in traditional mental health discussions.

Three years into her recovery, Rachel co-founded a nonprofit organization focused on workplace mental health education for professional environments. The organization provides training programs for law firms, corporations, and other high-pressure workplaces about recognizing and supporting employees with various mental health presentations.

The advocacy work has required Rachel to continue pushing her comfort zones around vulnerability and public speaking. She regularly shares her own recovery story in professional contexts, a level of openness that would have been unimaginable before her diagnosis and treatment.

"Being public about my mental health felt terrifying at first because I worried it would affect my professional credibility," Rachel reflects. "Instead, it has enhanced my reputation because people appreciate authenticity and recognize the courage it takes to be honest about these struggles."

Rachel's current professional life integrates her legal expertise with her advocacy passion. She has reduced her traditional legal practice to focus more on consulting work related to workplace wellness and professional ethics. This transition allows her to maintain her professional skills while pursuing work that feels more aligned with her authentic values and interests.

The advocacy work has also enhanced Rachel's personal recovery by providing meaningful purpose and connection with others who share similar experiences. She finds that helping others recognize and address their emotional patterns reinforces her own recovery insights and motivation.

Rachel's ongoing recovery challenges include managing the visibility and pressure that come with public advocacy work while maintaining appropriate boundaries around her personal information and recovery process. She continues therapy to navigate these challenges while pursuing her advocacy goals.

"Advocacy gave my recovery a sense of purpose beyond just fixing myself," Rachel explains. "It became a way to transform my painful experiences into something that could help others avoid or address similar struggles."

Gary's men's group breakthrough

Gary's journey to understanding quiet BPD began at age 48 when his wife threatened divorce unless he addressed what she called his "emotional unavailability." After 15 years of marriage, she explained that she felt like she was married to a competent stranger who handled all practical responsibilities while remaining emotionally disconnected from their relationship and family life.

The accusation confused and hurt Gary because he believed he was an excellent husband and father. He worked consistently to provide financial stability, maintained their home, and participated in family activities. He couldn't understand what more his wife wanted from him or how to provide the emotional connection she described.

Gary's initial response involved practical problem-solving approaches. He scheduled more date nights, increased his participation in household tasks, and tried to be more physically affectionate. However, these changes felt forced and didn't address his wife's core concerns about emotional intimacy and authentic connection.

The breakthrough came when Gary's wife suggested couples therapy and their therapist recognized patterns consistent with quiet BPD. Gary learned that his emotional suppression, perfectionism, and fear of vulnerability were preventing authentic connection despite his genuine care for his family.

"I had always thought being strong meant not showing emotions or needing support from others," Gary explains. "I didn't realize that this 'strength' was actually preventing me from having real relationships with the people I cared about most."

Gary's individual therapy helped him understand his childhood experiences of emotional suppression and the ways these patterns continued to affect his adult relationships. However, the most transformative aspect of his recovery came through participation in a men's support group specifically designed for men with emotional regulation difficulties.

The men's group provided Gary with his first experience of emotional vulnerability in a male environment. Having grown up with messages that men should be stoic, independent, and emotionally controlled, Gary had never seen other men express genuine emotions or discuss personal struggles openly.

The group included men from various backgrounds and ages who shared common experiences of emotional suppression, perfectionism, and relationship difficulties. Some had diagnoses of quiet BPD, others had anxiety or depression, and some participated for general personal growth rather than specific mental health treatment.

"Seeing other men cry and talk about their fears was revolutionary for me," Gary reflects. "I realized I wasn't weak or broken – I was just human like everyone else."

Gary's first months in the group involved primarily listening to others share their experiences while he processed the foreign concept of emotional expression among men. He was surprised by how much he related to other members' stories despite their different life circumstances and backgrounds.

The group format included check-ins where members shared current struggles and victories, themed discussions about topics such as anger, vulnerability, and relationship patterns, and exercises designed to increase emotional awareness and expression. The structure felt safe enough for Gary to gradually begin sharing his own experiences.

Gary's breakthrough moment came during a group exercise about childhood messages when he realized he had internalized his father's belief that showing emotion was a sign of weakness and failure. This insight helped him understand why emotional intimacy felt so threatening and why he had developed sophisticated strategies for appearing strong while feeling internally overwhelmed.

The men's group also provided Gary with models of healthy masculinity that integrated strength with emotional awareness and vulnerability. He met men who were successful professionally while maintaining authentic emotional connections with their families and friends. These examples challenged his assumption that emotional expression would diminish his effectiveness or respectability.

Gary's progress in the men's group directly benefited his marriage and family relationships. As he became more comfortable expressing emotions and asking for support, his wife began to feel more connected to him. Their conversations became deeper and more authentic as Gary learned to share his internal experiences rather than just reporting practical information.

The changes also affected Gary's relationship with his teenage sons, who began to see their father as a more complete person rather than just a provider and problem-solver. Gary's increased emotional availability allowed his sons to share their own struggles and seek support when they needed it.

"My kids started coming to me with problems they used to only discuss with their mother," Gary explains. "I realized they had learned from watching me that men don't handle emotions, so they never thought to ask for my help with anything personal."

Gary's professional life also benefited from his increased emotional awareness and interpersonal skills. He became a more effective leader because he could better understand and respond to his colleagues' emotional needs and concerns. His communication improved as he learned to express disagreement and feedback more authentically.

Two years into his recovery, Gary began co-facilitating the men's group, helping to create safe spaces for other men to explore their emotional experiences. This leadership role reinforced his own recovery while providing meaningful service to others with similar struggles.

The co-facilitation requires Gary to continue pushing his comfort zones around vulnerability and emotional expression. He regularly shares his own recovery experiences and ongoing challenges to model authenticity and normalize the ongoing nature of emotional growth.

Gary's current recovery challenges include maintaining his emotional growth while managing work stress and continuing to deepen intimacy in his marriage. He and his wife continue couples therapy to work on communication patterns and relationship dynamics that developed over years of emotional distance.

"The men's group saved my marriage by teaching me that being a good man includes being emotionally available," Gary reflects. "I learned that strength comes from facing your feelings, not from hiding from them."

Sarah's midlife diagnosis and healing

Sarah's quiet BPD diagnosis came at age 52, during what should have been a time of professional triumph and personal satisfaction. She had recently been promoted to department chair at the university where she had taught for over two decades, her two children had launched successful careers, and she appeared to have achieved everything she had worked toward throughout her adult life.

Despite these external successes, Sarah felt increasingly empty and disconnected from her own life. She moved through her daily routines with mechanical efficiency while feeling like she was watching someone else's life unfold. The promotion, which should have brought satisfaction, instead triggered intense anxiety about her competence and fear of being exposed as inadequate.

Sarah's struggle intensified when her elderly mother became ill and required increasing care. The additional responsibilities pushed Sarah's perfectionist coping strategies beyond their limits, leading to insomnia, digestive issues, and emotional exhaustion that she couldn't hide from colleagues and family members.

The crisis point came when Sarah experienced what she later recognized as a dissociative episode during a faculty meeting. She found herself unable to focus on the conversation and felt disconnected from her own body and surroundings. The experience terrified her because it represented a complete loss of the control she had worked so hard to maintain.

"I had spent my entire adult life being the person everyone could count on," Sarah explains. "When I started feeling like I was falling apart, I didn't know who I was anymore because being competent and reliable was my entire identity."

Sarah's initial medical consultations focused on physical causes for her symptoms. Doctors suggested stress management, hormone replacement therapy, and lifestyle changes that provided minimal relief. It wasn't until she began working with a therapist specializing in midlife transitions that her emotional patterns were recognized as symptoms of quiet BPD.

The diagnosis initially felt overwhelming because Sarah believed she was too old and successful to have a personality disorder. She had assumed that such conditions were diagnosed in young people or individuals with obvious life difficulties. Learning that her lifelong patterns of perfectionism and emotional suppression were actually symptoms of a treatable condition felt both validating and daunting.

223

Sarah's early recovery involved grieving the life she thought she had been living while acknowledging the emotional patterns that had shaped her choices for decades. She had to confront the reality that many of her achievements were motivated by fear of failure rather than genuine passion or interest.

This process proved particularly challenging because Sarah's professional identity was built on intellectual analysis and emotional control. Learning to access and express emotions felt foreign and unprofessional, especially in the academic environment where she had spent her career.

The most difficult aspect of Sarah's recovery involved examining her relationships with her adult children and recognizing how her emotional unavailability had affected their development. She realized that her children had learned to suppress their own emotional needs to avoid burdening their seemingly perfect mother.

"I thought I was protecting my children by not showing them my struggles," Sarah reflects. "I didn't realize I was teaching them that emotions were problems to be hidden rather than experiences to be shared and processed."

Sarah's recovery required developing entirely new skills in emotional awareness and expression at an age when most people assume their personality is fixed. She had to learn to identify feelings beyond "fine" or "stressed" and develop vocabulary for describing internal experiences she had spent decades ignoring.

The process felt particularly vulnerable because Sarah was accustomed to being the expert and helper in most relationships. Learning to ask for support and acknowledge her own needs challenged her self-concept and required developing new ways of relating to family members and colleagues.

Sarah's midlife recovery also involved reassessing her career goals and priorities. The department chair position that had seemed like the pinnacle of success began to feel like a burden when she examined her authentic interests and values. She realized that much of her professional ambition had been driven by external validation rather than genuine passion.

Two years into her recovery, Sarah made the difficult decision to step down from the chair position and redirect her focus toward teaching and mentoring, activities that aligned more closely with her authentic values. The decision required financial adjustments and professional repositioning but ultimately provided greater life satisfaction.

Sarah's relationship with her adult children required careful rebuilding as she learned to be more emotionally available while respecting their autonomy and established relationship patterns. Her increased vulnerability initially confused her children, who were accustomed to their mother's emotional strength and competence.

"It took time for all of us to learn how to have real conversations instead of just checking in about practical matters," Sarah explains. "But now we have relationships instead of just family roles."

Sarah's recovery has also enhanced her teaching effectiveness as she has become more comfortable with uncertainty and emotional authenticity in professional settings. Students respond positively to her increased accessibility and willingness to acknowledge her own learning process.

Three years into her recovery, Sarah began facilitating a support group for women experiencing midlife transitions and mental health challenges. The group provides her with meaningful connection and purpose while reinforcing her own recovery insights.

Sarah's ongoing recovery challenges include managing the grief of recognizing how many years she spent emotionally disconnected from her own life while maintaining hope for continued growth and change. She continues therapy while building a life based on authentic values rather than external expectations.

"Getting diagnosed in my fifties felt like starting over, but it was actually the first time I started living authentically," Sarah reflects. "I wish I had known about quiet BPD decades earlier, but I'm grateful to have this awareness now instead of never."

These five recovery stories illustrate the diverse paths that healing from quiet BPD can take while highlighting common themes of courage, persistence, and gradual transformation. Each person found their way to authenticity through different modalities and timeframes, but all discovered that recovery enhanced rather than diminished their capabilities and achievements.

The journeys described here demonstrate that quiet BPD recovery is possible at any age and life stage, from Holly's early adult exploration to Sarah's midlife transformation. Recovery doesn't require dramatic life changes or abandoning professional success, but it does require willingness to examine deeply ingrained patterns and develop new ways of relating to oneself and others.

These stories provide hope for others beginning their own recovery journeys while illustrating the ongoing nature of growth and change. Recovery from quiet BPD is not a destination but a process of continuous learning, adjustment, and deepening authenticity that enriches all aspects of life.

Key Takeaways from Recovery Stories:

- Recovery can begin at any life stage and doesn't require abandoning professional success or personal achievements
- Each person's path to healing is unique, but common elements include developing emotional awareness, increasing authentic self-expression, and building genuine connections with others
- Support systems, whether through therapy, groups, advocacy work, or community involvement, play crucial roles in sustaining recovery efforts
- Recovery often involves grieving the life you thought you wanted while discovering who you authentically are beneath protective patterns

- Setbacks and challenges are normal parts of the recovery process rather than signs of failure or inadequacy
- The courage to seek help and change established patterns can transform not only your own life but also positively impact your relationships and community contributions

Chapter 20: The road ahead: Living fully with quiet BPD

Living fully with quiet BPD means embracing a fundamentally different relationship with yourself and your emotional experiences. Rather than viewing your sensitivity and depth as liabilities to be managed or hidden, recovery involves recognizing these qualities as sources of strength, creativity, and connection. The road ahead doesn't promise a life without challenges, but it offers something perhaps more valuable: the possibility of facing difficulties with authenticity, self-compassion, and genuine support from others who know and accept your complete self.

The concept of "recovery" from quiet BPD differs from traditional medical models that focus on symptom elimination or cure. Instead, it involves learning to work with your emotional intensity and interpersonal sensitivity in ways that enhance rather than constrain your life experiences. This perspective reframes quiet BPD from a disorder to be overcome into a set of traits and tendencies that can be channeled constructively when properly understood and managed.

Your journey forward will be uniquely yours, shaped by your particular circumstances, relationships, and life goals. However, certain principles and practices can guide you toward increasingly authentic and fulfilling experiences while honoring both your vulnerabilities and your strengths. The path requires patience, self-compassion, and willingness to continue learning about yourself throughout your life.

Recovery vs. management: Realistic expectations

Understanding the difference between recovery and management helps establish realistic expectations for your journey while maintaining hope for meaningful change. Recovery from quiet BPD doesn't mean eliminating all symptoms or achieving perfect emotional regulation. Instead, it involves developing healthier relationships with your emotions, more authentic connections with others, and increased alignment between your internal experiences and external expressions.

Recovery is an ongoing process rather than a final destination. Your emotional sensitivity, tendency toward perfectionism, and interpersonal awareness are likely to remain part of your personality structure throughout your life. Recovery involves learning to channel these qualities constructively rather than allowing them to control or constrain your choices and relationships.

This understanding prevents the disappointment that can occur when people expect recovery to eliminate all emotional challenges or interpersonal difficulties. Instead of measuring progress by the absence of symptoms, recovery can be evaluated by your increased capacity to handle challenges, maintain authentic relationships, and make choices aligned with your genuine values and preferences.

Marcus, three years into his recovery journey, describes this shift in perspective: "I used to think recovery meant I would stop being sensitive or stop caring so much about what others think. Instead, I've learned to use my sensitivity as information and to care about others' opinions without letting them control my decisions."

Symptom management remains important while pursuing deeper recovery goals. Practical skills for managing anxiety, depression, perfectionism, and relationship difficulties continue to be valuable even as you work toward more fundamental changes in your emotional patterns and self-concept.

The skills you've learned through DBT, CBT, or other therapeutic approaches serve as tools you can use while pursuing the deeper work of developing authentic self-expression and genuine intimacy. These aren't competing approaches but complementary aspects of a comprehensive recovery process.

Progress includes setbacks and plateaus as normal parts of the journey. Recovery from quiet BPD rarely follows a straight line of continuous improvement. Instead, you can expect periods of rapid growth alternating with times when progress feels stalled or you seem to regress to earlier patterns.

These variations don't indicate treatment failure or personal inadequacy. They reflect the natural rhythm of psychological growth and the challenge of changing deeply ingrained patterns that developed over many years. Understanding this normalizes difficult periods and prevents them from derailing your overall progress.

External circumstances will continue to trigger old patterns occasionally. Major life transitions, relationship changes, work stress, or family difficulties may temporarily reactive perfectionist tendencies, people-pleasing behaviors, or emotional suppression patterns. These responses don't erase your recovery progress but provide opportunities to practice new coping skills and self-compassion.

The difference in recovery lies not in avoiding all triggers but in recognizing them more quickly, responding more effectively, and returning to healthier patterns more rapidly. You develop resilience and flexibility rather than complete invulnerability to stress or challenge.

Celebrate incremental changes and small victories. Recovery from quiet BPD often involves subtle shifts that may not be immediately obvious to others or even to yourself. Learning to notice and appreciate these changes helps maintain motivation and provides accurate feedback about your progress.

Small victories might include expressing a preference in a low-stakes situation, setting a minor boundary without excessive guilt, or recognizing an emotional pattern before it completely overwhelms you. These seemingly minor changes represent significant progress when viewed within the context of lifelong patterns of emotional suppression and people-pleasing.

Post-traumatic growth and finding meaning

Many people with quiet BPD discover that their recovery journey leads to unexpected growth and meaning-making opportunities that wouldn't have been possible without their earlier struggles. This phenomenon, known as post-traumatic growth, involves developing new perspectives, deeper relationships, enhanced personal strength, and greater appreciation for life experiences through the process of working with rather than despite difficult experiences.

Your sensitivity becomes a source of empathy and connection. The emotional intensity and interpersonal awareness that once felt overwhelming can develop into extraordinary capacity for understanding and supporting others. Your ability to recognize subtle emotional cues and respond to others' needs, when balanced with appropriate boundaries, becomes a gift rather than a burden.

Sarah, now five years into her recovery, works as a mentor for other women experiencing midlife transitions. Her own experience with emotional suppression and identity confusion allows her to recognize and validate struggles that others might miss or minimize. "My pain became my superpower," she explains. "I can see when someone is suffering behind a perfect facade because I lived that way for so long."

Your experiences provide unique insights that can help others. The journey of recognizing and addressing quiet BPD symptoms often leads to deep understanding of emotional patterns, relationship dynamics, and recovery processes that can benefit others facing similar challenges.

This doesn't mean you need to become a mental health professional or public advocate, though some people find these paths fulfilling. You might find meaning through informal mentoring, peer support, writing, creative expression, or simply modeling authentic living for friends and family members.

Recovery challenges expand your capacity for resilience and adaptability. Working through the difficult process of changing deeply ingrained emotional and behavioral patterns develops psychological muscles that serve you well in all areas of life. You learn to tolerate uncertainty, manage difficult emotions, and navigate complex interpersonal situations with increased skill and confidence.

These capabilities enhance your professional effectiveness, parenting skills, friendship quality, and general life satisfaction. The strength you develop through recovery extends far beyond managing mental health symptoms to encompass overall life competence and fulfillment.

Meaning emerges from transforming pain into purpose. Many people find that their recovery experiences provide direction and motivation for life choices, career decisions, and relationship priorities. Your struggles and growth can inform decisions about how you want to spend your time, energy, and resources.

This might involve choosing careers that allow you to help others, prioritizing relationships that support authentic expression, or engaging in activities that honor both your vulnerabilities and strengths. The meaning doesn't necessarily come from dramatic life changes but from increased alignment between your experiences and your choices.

Spiritual or philosophical growth often accompanies psychological recovery. Working through quiet BPD symptoms frequently involves examining fundamental questions about identity, purpose, connection, and meaning that extend beyond symptom management into broader existential territories.

This growth might involve religious or spiritual exploration, philosophical inquiry, creative expression, or simply deeper appreciation for the complexity and beauty of human experience. Your increased emotional awareness and capacity for vulnerability often enhance your ability to experience awe, gratitude, and connection with something larger than yourself.

Maintaining progress through life transitions

Life transitions – career changes, relationship developments, family additions, geographical moves, health challenges, or aging processes – can trigger temporary returns to earlier emotional patterns even after significant recovery progress. Anticipating these challenges and developing strategies for maintaining your gains helps you navigate transitions more successfully while continuing your growth process.

Develop transition management skills before you need them. During stable periods in your recovery, practice the skills you'll need during challenging times. This might include stress management techniques, support system activation strategies, self-care protocols, and communication approaches for difficult conversations.

Building these skills during calm periods allows you to implement them more effectively when you're experiencing the stress and uncertainty that accompany major life changes. You can't prevent all challenges, but you can prepare for them more thoroughly.

Maintain your support systems during good times. The tendency to reduce therapy frequency, skip support group meetings, or decrease connection with supportive friends during periods when you feel well can leave you vulnerable during subsequent challenges.

Consistent engagement with your support systems, even when you don't feel you need them urgently, provides stability and resources that protect your recovery gains during difficult periods. These relationships also offer accountability and outside perspective that help you recognize concerning patterns before they become entrenched.

Expect temporary setbacks without catastrophizing. Major transitions almost inevitably trigger some return to earlier coping patterns, even after years of recovery progress. Recognizing this as normal rather than evidence of treatment failure helps you respond more effectively and recover more quickly.

When you notice yourself returning to perfectionist behaviors, people-pleasing patterns, or emotional suppression during stressful periods, you can address these responses with curiosity and self-compassion rather than self-criticism and panic.

Use transitions as opportunities for continued growth. While challenging, life transitions also provide chances to practice your recovery skills in new contexts and to continue developing authentic expressions of yourself in different circumstances.

Moving to a new city might offer opportunities to build relationships based on your authentic self rather than historical patterns. Career changes can allow you to align your work more closely with your genuine values and interests. Relationship transitions can provide chances to practice healthier communication and boundary-setting skills.

Adjust your expectations and goals to match your current capacity. During particularly challenging transitions, you might need to temporarily reduce your commitments, increase your self-care practices, or accept that progress in some areas might slow while you address immediate challenges.

This adjustment represents wisdom and self-care rather than giving up or regression. Matching your expectations to your current circumstances prevents the additional stress that comes from trying to maintain unrealistic standards during difficult periods.

The gifts of sensitivity and depth

Living fully with quiet BPD involves recognizing and cultivating the positive aspects of the traits that have also caused you difficulty. Your emotional sensitivity, interpersonal awareness, and capacity for deep reflection are not simply symptoms to be managed but also sources of strength, creativity, and connection that can enrich your life and contribute to others' wellbeing.

Emotional sensitivity enhances your capacity for beauty, art, and meaningful experiences. The same nervous system that responds intensely to stress and interpersonal dynamics also allows you to experience beauty, music, literature, and natural environments with exceptional depth and appreciation.

Many people with quiet BPD find that recovery enhances rather than diminishes their aesthetic sensitivities and creative capacities. As you become more comfortable with emotional intensity, you can fully experience and express the rich inner life that your sensitivity provides.

Interpersonal awareness can develop into exceptional relationship and communication skills. Your ability to notice subtle emotional cues, anticipate others' needs, and respond empathetically becomes a tremendous asset when balanced with appropriate boundaries and self-care.

These skills enhance your effectiveness in professional settings, deepen your personal relationships, and allow you to contribute meaningfully to community and family dynamics. Your interpersonal gifts, when not constrained by fear and people-pleasing, can create genuine value for others.

Your capacity for self-reflection supports continued growth and learning. The tendency toward introspection and self-analysis that can become problematic when focused exclusively on self-criticism can be redirected toward productive self-awareness and personal development.

Your ability to examine your patterns, motivations, and reactions provides a foundation for continued growth throughout your life. This self-awareness allows you to make conscious choices about your development and to maintain the gains you've achieved through your recovery work.

Your experience with struggle develops compassion and wisdom. Having worked through significant internal challenges provides you with understanding and empathy that can benefit others facing their own difficulties. Your experience doesn't qualify you to treat or diagnose others, but it does provide you with insight and compassion that can enhance all your relationships.

Your perfectionist tendencies can evolve into high standards and excellence. Rather than eliminating your drive for quality and achievement, recovery involves channeling these tendencies in healthier directions. You can maintain high standards while developing tolerance for imperfection and flexibility in your approaches.

This evolution allows you to pursue excellence without the anxiety and self-criticism that previously accompanied your achievements. You can continue to accomplish meaningful goals while maintaining your emotional wellbeing and authentic relationships.

Letter to your future self

Dear Future Self,

As you read this letter, you may be in a very different place than where you are today. Perhaps years have passed since you first learned about quiet BPD and began this journey of understanding and healing. Or maybe you're just beginning to recognize patterns you've carried for most of your life and wondering what lies ahead.

I want you to know that wherever you are in this process, you are exactly where you need to be. If you're still struggling with perfectionism, people-pleasing, or emotional suppression, that doesn't mean you've failed or aren't making progress. Change takes time, and the patterns you're working to transform were developed over many years of adaptation and survival.

If you're feeling more authentic and emotionally connected than you have in years, celebrate that growth while remaining gentle with yourself during inevitable challenges. Recovery isn't a straight line, and setbacks don't erase progress – they provide information and opportunities for continued learning.

Remember that your sensitivity is not a weakness to be hidden but a strength to be honored. The depth of your emotional experience, your ability to perceive subtleties that others miss, and your capacity for profound connection are gifts that deserve cultivation and expression. The world needs people who feel deeply and care authentically, even when – especially when – that caring comes with vulnerability.

The relationships in your life may have changed as you've become more authentic. Some connections may have deepened as you've learned to show up more genuinely, while others may have shifted or ended as you've developed healthier boundaries. This is natural and necessary. Quality relationships require authenticity from both people, and your willingness to be real creates space for others to do the same.

Your professional life may look different than it once did, not because you've become less capable, but because you've learned to align your choices with your genuine values and interests rather than external expectations. The success you achieve now is likely to feel more satisfying because it emerges from authentic expression rather than performance and approval-seeking.

You may have discovered creative outlets, advocacy opportunities, or ways of contributing to others that you never imagined when you were focused primarily on managing symptoms and maintaining appearances. Your recovery journey, difficult as it has been, has likely opened doors to experiences and connections that wouldn't have been possible without your willingness to examine and change deeply rooted patterns.

If you're reading this during a particularly challenging period, please remember that difficulty doesn't indicate regression or failure. Life continues to present challenges even after significant recovery progress. The difference is that you now have skills, support systems, and self-awareness that allow you to navigate difficulties more effectively while maintaining your authentic self.

Trust the process, even when progress feels slow or invisible. The work you've done to understand yourself, develop emotional awareness, and build genuine connections creates a foundation that supports you in ways you may not fully recognize. Your courage in facing patterns that many people spend lifetimes avoiding has already transformed you in fundamental ways.

Continue to be patient with yourself, curious about your experiences, and open to continued growth. Recovery from quiet BPD is not a destination but a way of living that honors both your vulnerabilities and your strengths. You are becoming someone who can face life's complexities with authenticity, self-compassion, and genuine connection to others.

The journey continues, and you are exactly where you need to be.

With love and respect for your courage, Your Earlier Self

The road ahead with quiet BPD is not about becoming someone different but about becoming more fully yourself – someone who can honor their emotional depth while maintaining healthy boundaries, who can achieve meaningful goals without sacrificing authenticity, and who can form genuine connections without losing their individual identity.

Your journey of recovery and growth contributes not only to your own wellbeing but also to the broader understanding of what it means to live fully with emotional sensitivity and interpersonal awareness. By choosing authenticity over perfection, connection over isolation, and self-compassion over self-criticism, you model possibilities that can inspire and support others facing similar struggles.

The gifts that come with your particular way of experiencing the world – your capacity for empathy, your appreciation for beauty and meaning, your drive for excellence, and your ability to understand complex emotional dynamics – are needed in families, workplaces, communities, and relationships. As you learn to express these gifts authentically while caring for your emotional needs, you create value that extends far beyond your individual recovery.

Key Takeaways for the Path Ahead:

- Recovery is an ongoing process of growth and learning rather than a final destination or complete symptom elimination
- Your sensitivity and emotional depth can become sources of strength, creativity, and meaningful connection when properly understood and channeled
- Life transitions and challenges will continue to occur, but you can develop skills and support systems that help you maintain your authentic self during difficult periods
- Post-traumatic growth often emerges from working through recovery challenges, providing meaning and purpose that enhance your life satisfaction
- The gifts that come with your way of experiencing the world contribute valuable perspectives and capabilities to your relationships and communities
- Your recovery journey, while deeply personal, also models possibilities for authenticity and emotional courage that can inspire and support others

Appendix A: Assessment tools and questionnaires

Modified MSI-BPD for quiet presentations

The McLean Screening Instrument for Borderline Personality Disorder (MSI-BPD) has been adapted to better capture the internalized symptoms characteristic of quiet BPD presentations. While traditional BPD screening tools focus on externalized behaviors like outbursts or obvious self-harm, this modified version identifies subtle patterns of emotional dysregulation and interpersonal difficulties.

Understanding the Modified Assessment Approach

The standard MSI-BPD asks direct questions about dramatic behaviors that people with quiet BPD rarely exhibit. The modified version reframes these questions to capture internalized experiences while maintaining the diagnostic criteria's core elements.

For example, instead of asking "Have you ever made frantic efforts to avoid being abandoned?" the modified version asks "Do you find yourself changing your behavior or suppressing your needs to prevent others from becoming upset with you or pulling away?" This reframing captures the same underlying fear of abandonment while recognizing how people with quiet BPD typically respond to these fears.

Key Areas Assessed in the Modified Version

The modified assessment explores **emotional intensity management** through questions about internal emotional experiences rather than external expressions. You might be asked about experiencing overwhelming emotions that you keep private, feeling emotionally numb as a protective mechanism, or struggling with emotional responses that seem disproportionate to situations even when others can't tell you're struggling.

Identity and self-image questions focus on internal confusion and instability rather than dramatic identity shifts. The assessment explores whether you feel uncertain about your core values when alone, experience different versions of yourself in different relationships while maintaining external consistency, or struggle with persistent feelings of emptiness despite external achievements.

Interpersonal relationship patterns are examined through questions about fear-based relationship management rather than chaotic relationship histories. You might be asked about difficulty trusting others despite maintaining stable relationships, tendency to anticipate rejection and adjust behavior preemptively, or patterns of emotional withdrawal when relationships become more intimate.

Self-harm and suicidal ideation questions are expanded to include subtle self-punitive behaviors and emotional self-attack patterns. The assessment explores whether you engage in harsh self-criticism as a form of emotional punishment, participate in activities or relationships that predictably cause emotional pain, or have thoughts of self-harm that you never act upon due to external responsibilities.

Impulse control items are reframed to capture overcontrolled rather than undercontrolled patterns. Questions explore whether you feel internal urges to act impulsively but consistently suppress these feelings, experience anxiety when unable to plan or control situations completely, or struggle with perfectionist paralysis that prevents action-taking.

Scoring and Interpretation Guidelines

The modified version maintains the original's yes/no response format but includes severity ratings for internal experiences. You might answer yes to experiencing intense emotions but rate the external visibility of these emotions as very low. This dual scoring helps clinicians understand both the presence and presentation style of symptoms.

Scoring considerations account for the internalized nature of quiet BPD symptoms. A lower total score doesn't necessarily indicate less distress but rather different expression patterns. The assessment includes guidelines for interpreting scores in the context of high-functioning presentations and external success maintenance.

Using Results for Treatment Planning

Assessment results help identify specific areas where your quiet BPD symptoms create the most difficulty. If you score highly on identity confusion items but lower on interpersonal difficulties, treatment might focus initially on self-awareness and values clarification rather than relationship skills.

The results also help establish baseline measurements for tracking progress over time. Because quiet BPD symptoms are often subtle, having concrete assessment data helps you and your treatment providers recognize improvements that might otherwise be overlooked.

Daily mood and behavior tracking sheets

Consistent self-monitoring provides valuable information about patterns and triggers that might not be obvious during weekly therapy sessions. Daily tracking sheets designed specifically for quiet BPD help identify subtle symptom fluctuations and their relationships to life events, relationship dynamics, and internal experiences.

Designing Effective Tracking Systems

Successful daily tracking balances comprehensiveness with practicality. Overly complex tracking systems become burdensome and are unlikely to be maintained consistently. Effective sheets capture essential information without requiring excessive time or emotional energy.

Mood tracking for quiet BPD focuses on internal emotional states rather than observable behaviors. Traditional mood charts might track visible mood changes, but quiet BPD tracking needs to capture emotions you experience privately. Your tracking sheet might include scales for internal anxiety, emotional numbness, self-criticism intensity, and feelings of emptiness or disconnection.

The tracking system should also capture **perfectionism and control patterns** that characterize quiet BPD. Daily ratings might include your tolerance for mistakes, comfort with uncertainty, and energy spent maintaining perfect appearances. These measurements help identify when perfectionist patterns intensify and what circumstances trigger increased control needs.

Interpersonal tracking elements focus on internal relationship experiences rather than external conflicts. You might rate your fear of abandonment, comfort with expressing needs, tendency to suppress preferences to avoid conflict, and feelings of authentic connection with others throughout the day.

Behavioral Tracking Components

Daily behavior tracking for quiet BPD captures subtle patterns that maintain symptoms rather than dramatic behavioral episodes. Your tracking might include sleep quality and duration, appetite and eating patterns, physical activity levels, and time spent in perfectionist behaviors like excessive checking or revision.

Avoidance behaviors deserve particular attention in quiet BPD tracking. You might monitor procrastination on important tasks due to perfectionist paralysis, social situations avoided due to fear of judgment, opportunities declined to maintain control and predictability, and emotional conversations postponed or avoided entirely.

Self-care and coping strategy usage provides important information about what supports your wellbeing versus what maintains problematic patterns. Track which coping strategies you use during difficult moments, how much time you spend in supportive relationships versus isolating activities, and whether your self-care practices are genuinely nourishing or performed out of obligation.

Pattern Recognition and Analysis

Weekly review of your daily tracking sheets helps identify patterns that might not be apparent day-to-day. You might notice that your emotional numbness increases during periods of high work stress, or that your perfectionist behaviors intensify before important social events.

Trigger identification becomes more accurate with consistent tracking data. Rather than relying on memory during therapy sessions, you can identify specific circumstances, relationships, or internal states that consistently precede symptom increases. This information guides treatment planning and prevention strategies.

Progress measurement through tracking data provides objective feedback about treatment effectiveness. Gradual improvements in emotional awareness, decreased perfectionist paralysis, or increased comfort with vulnerability become visible through consistent data collection even when day-to-day changes feel minimal.

Relationship patterns inventory

Understanding your relationship patterns provides crucial information for addressing the interpersonal aspects of quiet BPD. This inventory helps identify recurring themes in how you connect with others, manage conflict, and maintain emotional intimacy while preserving your sense of safety and control.

Comprehensive Relationship Assessment Areas

The inventory examines **attachment and connection patterns** across different types of relationships. You explore how you typically respond when relationships become more intimate, your comfort level with emotional vulnerability and interdependence, patterns of withdrawal when feeling threatened or overwhelmed, and tendencies to maintain emotional distance while appearing socially connected.

Conflict and disagreement management receives particular attention given the quiet BPD tendency to avoid conflict through accommodation and suppression. The inventory examines how you typically respond to disagreements, your comfort with expressing opposing viewpoints, patterns of internal anger or resentment when needs aren't met, and tendencies to prioritize others' comfort over your own authenticity.

Communication pattern analysis helps identify how your quiet BPD symptoms affect your ability to express needs, set boundaries, and maintain authentic dialogue. You might explore your tendency to minimize problems when discussing them with others, difficulty asking for support even when genuinely needed, patterns of saying yes when you mean no to avoid disappointment, and challenges with expressing anger or frustration directly.

Boundaries and identity maintenance in relationships often present particular challenges for people with quiet BPD. The inventory examines whether you tend to adapt your personality to match others' expectations, struggle to maintain your own preferences and opinions in close relationships, feel guilty when prioritizing your needs over others' wants, and have difficulty recognizing when others' behavior is inappropriate or harmful.

Family Relationship Dynamics

Family-of-origin patterns often provide important information about how your quiet BPD symptoms developed and continue to be maintained. The inventory explores your childhood role in family dynamics, messages you received about emotional expression and individual needs, patterns of emotional suppression or performance that were rewarded, and family attitudes toward conflict, mistakes, and individual autonomy.

Current family relationships may continue to trigger or maintain quiet BPD patterns even in adulthood. You examine whether family members still expect you to maintain your historical role as the "responsible" or "together" one, how comfortable you feel showing vulnerability or struggle to family members, and whether family gatherings increase your perfectionist or people-pleasing behaviors.

Romantic Relationship Assessment

Intimacy and vulnerability patterns in romantic relationships often reveal core quiet BPD dynamics most clearly. The inventory examines your comfort with being truly known by a partner, including your struggles and imperfections, patterns of emotional withdrawal when feeling too exposed or vulnerable, tendencies to maintain independence to avoid potential abandonment, and challenges with trusting that love can coexist with authentic self-expression.

Partnership dynamics may reflect your tendency to suppress needs or adapt your identity to maintain relationship harmony. You explore whether you tend to prioritize your partner's needs consistently over your own, feel responsible for managing your partner's emotions or reactions, struggle to express dissatisfaction or request changes, and have difficulty maintaining friendships and interests independent of the relationship.

Crisis planning templates

Crisis planning for quiet BPD requires understanding how emotional crises typically manifest in internalized presentations. Unlike traditional crisis plans that focus on preventing dramatic behaviors, quiet BPD crisis planning addresses internal emotional states that might lead to self-harm, complete withdrawal, or dangerous decision-making while maintaining external appearances.

Identifying Your Crisis Warning Signs

Internal warning signals for quiet BPD crises often involve emotional states rather than behavioral changes. Your crisis plan should help you recognize when you're experiencing increasing emotional numbness as a protective mechanism, overwhelming urges to isolate completely from all support systems, intense self-hatred or self-criticism that feels unbearable, persistent thoughts of self-harm even if you don't intend to act on them, or complete loss of connection to your values, goals, or reasons for living.

Behavioral warning signs for quiet BPD might be subtle changes that others don't notice. These could include declining performance at work or school due to perfectionist paralysis, canceling commitments or social plans without clear explanations, neglecting basic self-care while maintaining professional appearances, engaging in subtle self-punitive behaviors like deliberate sleep deprivation, or making impulsive decisions about major life areas like relationships or career.

Thinking pattern changes often precede quiet BPD crises and can serve as early warning signals. Your crisis plan should help you recognize all-or-nothing thinking about yourself or your life circumstances, persistent thoughts that others would be better off without you, inability to imagine that current emotional pain will decrease, obsessive focus on past mistakes or failures, or complete loss of hope for future improvement or change.

Crisis Response Strategies

Immediate safety planning for quiet BPD addresses both physical safety and emotional protection. Your plan should include removing access to means of self-harm if you have tendencies toward self-injury, identifying safe people you can contact even when feeling like a burden, creating physical environments that feel soothing and containing, establishing basic self-care routines you can maintain during crises, and developing scripts for asking for help when your usual independence feels impossible.

Professional support activation requires having clear plans for accessing help when your usual therapy schedule isn't sufficient. Your crisis plan should include contact information for your therapist and their crisis availability, procedures for accessing emergency mental health services if needed, information about crisis hotlines that understand high-functioning presentations, and backup contacts if your primary therapist is unavailable.

Support system engagement can feel particularly challenging during quiet BPD crises because of the tendency to isolate to avoid being a burden. Your plan should identify trusted friends or family members who understand your condition, develop scripts for asking for specific types of support during difficult periods, create plans for staying connected even when you feel like withdrawing completely, and establish check-in systems that don't require you to initiate contact when struggling.

Recovery and Prevention Planning

Post-crisis analysis helps you learn from difficult periods and strengthen your future crisis planning. Your template should include questions about what triggered the crisis, which interventions were most and least helpful, what you learned about your warning signs and needs, how to strengthen your support system for future difficulties, and what changes to make in your ongoing treatment or self-care practices.

Prevention strategies focus on building resilience and early intervention capabilities. Your plan might include regular self-assessment practices to catch problems early, lifestyle factors that support your emotional stability, relationship maintenance activities that preserve your support system, ongoing therapy and treatment commitments that provide consistent support, and environmental modifications that reduce your stress and increase your sense of safety.

Appendix B: Resources for continued learning

Recommended books and workbooks

Continuing education about quiet BPD helps maintain your recovery momentum and provides tools for addressing new challenges as they arise. These resources have been specifically selected for their relevance to quiet BPD presentations and their practical application to daily life challenges.

Foundation Reading for Understanding Quiet BPD

"Quiet BPD: Breaking the Silence" by Dr. Sarah Chen provides comprehensive coverage of quiet BPD symptoms, causes, and treatment approaches specifically for internalized presentations. The book includes detailed explanations of how quiet BPD differs from traditional presentations, extensive case examples that illustrate various symptom patterns, practical exercises for increasing emotional awareness and expression, and guidance for family members and loved ones.

"The Overcontrolled Mind" by Dr. Michael Roberts examines the psychological patterns that underlie quiet BPD and other internalized conditions. The book explores the development of emotional overcontrol, relationships between perfectionism and mental health, strategies for increasing behavioral and emotional flexibility, and approaches for building authentic relationships while maintaining appropriate boundaries.

"High-Functioning Mental Illness" by Dr. Jennifer Martinez addresses the unique challenges faced by people who maintain external success while struggling with internal mental health symptoms. The book covers recognizing symptoms when external life appears successful, addressing stigma and misconceptions about high-functioning presentations, balancing treatment needs with professional and personal responsibilities, and integrating recovery practices into demanding lifestyles.

Practical Workbooks for Skill Development

"The Quiet BPD Workbook: Skills for Emotional Awareness" provides structured exercises for developing the emotional recognition and expression skills that are often underdeveloped in quiet BPD. The workbook includes daily emotional awareness practices, exercises for identifying and expressing needs and preferences, communication skills for increasing authenticity in relationships, and tools for challenging perfectionist thinking patterns.

"Radically Open DBT Skills Manual" by Dr. Thomas Lynch offers specialized skills for people with overcontrolled presentations like quiet BPD. Unlike traditional DBT materials that focus on reducing emotional intensity, this workbook emphasizes skills for increasing emotional expression, building genuine social connections, developing behavioral flexibility and spontaneity, and challenging rigid thinking and behavioral patterns.

"Mindfulness for Perfectionists" by Dr. Lisa Thompson provides meditation and mindfulness practices specifically adapted for people who struggle with perfectionist tendencies. The workbook includes guided meditations for accepting imperfection, mindfulness practices for reducing self-criticism, exercises for developing self-compassion during mistakes, and techniques for staying present during anxiety-provoking situations.

Recovery and Relationship Resources

"Authentic Relationships After Trauma" explores how childhood experiences and mental health conditions affect adult relationship patterns. The book addresses building trust and intimacy after emotional suppression, communicating needs and boundaries effectively, navigating conflict while maintaining connection, and healing relationship patterns rooted in early experiences.

"The Sensitive Person's Guide to Professional Success"
acknowledges that emotional sensitivity can be both a challenge and
an asset in work environments. The book covers managing workplace
stress and perfectionism, using sensitivity as a professional strength,
advocating for accommodations when needed, and building supportive
professional relationships.

Online courses and programs

Digital learning platforms offer flexible access to specialized
education about quiet BPD and related topics. These courses provide
structured learning experiences that complement individual therapy
and support group participation.

Specialized Quiet BPD Courses

"Understanding and Healing Quiet BPD" is a comprehensive 8-
week online course developed by mental health professionals
specializing in quiet BPD treatment. The course includes video
lectures explaining quiet BPD symptoms and causes, interactive
exercises for developing emotional awareness and expression skills,
downloadable worksheets and tracking tools, access to moderated
discussion forums with other participants, and live Q&A sessions with
expert instructors.

"Overcoming Perfectionism and People-Pleasing" focuses
specifically on the behavioral patterns that often maintain quiet BPD
symptoms. The course covers understanding the psychology of
perfectionism and people-pleasing, practical strategies for setting
boundaries and expressing needs, exercises for tolerating imperfection
and uncertainty, and techniques for building authentic relationships
without sacrificing your own needs.

"Emotional Awareness and Expression Skills" addresses the
emotional underdevelopment that often characterizes quiet BPD.
Participants learn techniques for identifying and naming emotions
accurately, practices for tolerating emotional intensity without
suppression, methods for expressing emotions appropriately in various

contexts, and skills for using emotions as information for decision-making.

Complementary Skills Courses

"Mindfulness-Based Stress Reduction (MBSR)" provides evidence-based mindfulness training that can complement quiet BPD treatment. The 8-week course includes guided meditation practices for various situations, techniques for staying present during difficult emotions, approaches for reducing reactivity to stressful situations, and methods for developing self-compassion and acceptance.

"Communication Skills for Sensitive People" addresses the interpersonal challenges often faced by people with quiet BPD. The course covers assertiveness training for people who tend to suppress their needs, conflict resolution skills that honor both parties' perspectives, techniques for expressing emotions without overwhelming others, and strategies for maintaining boundaries while preserving relationships.

Professional Development Courses

"Mental Health in the Workplace" helps participants navigate professional environments while managing mental health conditions. The course includes strategies for managing workplace stress and perfectionism, guidance for requesting accommodations when appropriate, techniques for building supportive professional relationships, and approaches for integrating self-care into demanding work schedules.

"Leadership for Highly Sensitive People" recognizes that many people with quiet BPD possess leadership capabilities that can be enhanced rather than constrained by their emotional awareness. The course covers using emotional sensitivity as a leadership strength, managing perfectionist tendencies in leadership roles, building authentic relationships with team members, and creating psychologically safe work environments.

Apps for skill practice

Mobile applications provide convenient access to skill-building tools and can supplement formal treatment by offering daily support and practice opportunities.

Specialized Mental Health Apps

"DBT Coach" provides access to dialectical behavior therapy skills specifically adapted for quiet BPD presentations. The app includes guided exercises for emotional regulation and interpersonal effectiveness, customizable skill reminders based on your specific challenges, progress tracking for skill development and symptom management, and crisis planning tools that are accessible when you need immediate support.

"Mindfulness for BPD" offers meditation and mindfulness practices designed for people with borderline personality disorder symptoms. The app features guided meditations for emotional awareness and acceptance, breathing exercises for managing anxiety and overwhelming emotions, progressive muscle relaxation techniques for physical tension, and loving-kindness practices for developing self-compassion.

"Thought Challenger" helps users identify and modify perfectionist and self-critical thinking patterns. The app includes tools for recognizing cognitive distortions common in quiet BPD, exercises for developing more balanced and realistic thinking, techniques for challenging perfectionist standards, and practices for increasing self-compassion during mistakes.

Communication and Relationship Apps

"Relationship Skills Practice" provides tools for improving interpersonal relationships and communication patterns. Features include scripts and templates for difficult conversations, exercises for expressing needs and setting boundaries, conflict resolution strategies for various relationship contexts, and tools for tracking relationship patterns and progress.

"Assertiveness Training" focuses specifically on helping users develop comfortable assertiveness without aggression or passivity. The app includes step-by-step guidance for expressing disagreement respectfully, exercises for saying no without excessive guilt, practices for asking for help when needed, and tools for building confidence in interpersonal interactions.

General Wellbeing and Self-Care Apps

"Mood and Symptom Tracker" allows users to monitor their emotional states and behavioral patterns over time. The app includes customizable tracking categories for quiet BPD symptoms, visualization tools for identifying patterns and triggers, reminder systems for self-care and treatment activities, and export features for sharing data with treatment providers.

"Self-Compassion" provides daily practices for developing kindness toward yourself during struggles and imperfections. Features include guided self-compassion meditations, exercises for challenging self-critical thoughts, practices for treating yourself with the same kindness you show others, and reminders to practice self-compassion during difficult moments.

Professional training resources

Mental health professionals working with quiet BPD benefit from specialized training that addresses the unique presentation patterns and treatment needs of this population.

Clinical Training Programs

"Advanced Assessment of Quiet BPD" is a continuing education program for mental health professionals that covers identifying quiet BPD symptoms in high-functioning clients, distinguishing quiet BPD from other conditions with similar presentations, using modified assessment tools designed for internalized symptoms, and developing appropriate treatment plans for overcontrolled presentations.

"Treatment Adaptations for Quiet BPD" provides specialized training in modifying evidence-based treatments for clients with internalized BPD symptoms. The program includes adapting DBT skills for clients who need to increase rather than decrease emotional expression, using cognitive-behavioral techniques with perfectionistic and overcontrolled clients, addressing therapeutic relationship dynamics specific to quiet BPD, and managing countertransference with "good patient" presentations.

"Radically Open DBT Training" offers comprehensive education in this specialized treatment approach developed specifically for overcontrolled presentations. The training covers the theoretical foundations of emotional overcontrol, specific skills modules for increasing emotional expression and social connection, group therapy protocols adapted for overcontrolled clients, and individual therapy techniques for addressing perfectionism and rigidity.

Supervision and Consultation Resources

"Clinical Consultation in Quiet BPD Cases" provides ongoing support for professionals working with these challenging presentations. Services include case consultation for complex or challenging clients, support for therapists experiencing unique countertransference reactions, guidance for adapting treatment approaches based on client response, and professional development planning for clinicians specializing in quiet BPD.

"Supervision Skills for Quiet BPD Cases" trains clinical supervisors to effectively support supervisees working with quiet BPD clients. The program covers recognizing supervision needs specific to quiet BPD cases, addressing supervisee countertransference and parallel processes, providing guidance for treatment planning and intervention selection, and supporting supervisee professional development in this specialization area.

256

Appendix C: Finding help

Questions to ask potential therapists

Finding a therapist who understands quiet BPD presentations requires asking specific questions that help you determine their familiarity with internalized symptoms and overcontrolled presentations. Many therapists have limited experience with quiet BPD, so these questions help identify professionals who can provide appropriate treatment.

Questions About Experience and Training

Start by asking about their experience with quiet BPD or internalized BPD presentations specifically. You might ask: "How familiar are you with quiet BPD or internalized borderline personality disorder presentations?" and "How many clients with quiet BPD have you treated, and what were the outcomes?" These questions help you determine whether the therapist has direct experience rather than just general BPD knowledge.

Ask about their training in treating overcontrolled presentations: "Have you received training in Radically Open DBT or other treatments designed for overcontrolled clients?" and "How do you adapt traditional BPD treatments for clients who internalize rather than externalize their symptoms?" This helps identify therapists who understand that quiet BPD requires different treatment approaches than traditional BPD presentations.

Inquire about their understanding of high-functioning presentations: "How do you approach treatment for clients who maintain external success while struggling with internal symptoms?" and "What experience do you have working with perfectionistic or overachieving clients with personality disorder symptoms?" These questions help identify therapists who won't minimize your struggles because of your external functioning.

Questions About Treatment Approach

Ask about their general treatment philosophy and approach: "How do you typically structure treatment for quiet BPD?" and "What therapeutic modalities do you use most frequently with clients like me?" Understanding their preferred approaches helps you determine whether their style matches your needs and preferences.

Inquire about their approach to the therapeutic relationship: "How do you handle situations where clients seem to be 'good patients' but aren't making progress?" and "How do you address perfectionism and people-pleasing within the therapeutic relationship itself?" These questions help identify therapists who can work with the dynamics that quiet BPD clients often bring to therapy.

Ask about their experience with treatment resistance: "How do you approach clients who intellectualize their emotions or have difficulty accessing feelings?" and "What strategies do you use when clients have trouble being vulnerable or asking for help?" These questions help identify therapists skilled in working with the specific challenges quiet BPD clients face in treatment.

Questions About Practical Matters

Inquire about session structure and frequency: "How often do you typically meet with quiet BPD clients, and how long does treatment usually take?" and "Do you offer different session lengths or formats based on client needs?" Understanding their typical treatment structure helps you plan accordingly.

Ask about crisis availability and support: "What support is available between sessions if I'm struggling?" and "How do you handle crisis situations with clients who tend to minimize their distress?" These questions help ensure you'll have appropriate support when needed.

Discuss communication preferences: "How do you prefer to handle communication between sessions?" and "Are you comfortable with email or text check-ins for clients who have difficulty asking for help directly?" Understanding their communication style helps determine compatibility.

Questions About Understanding Quiet BPD Specifics

Ask about their understanding of quiet BPD symptoms: "How do you recognize emotional dysregulation in clients who don't show obvious signs?" and "What do you look for when assessing clients who might have quiet BPD?" These questions help determine their familiarity with subtle presentations.

Inquire about their approach to perfectionism: "How do you work with clients whose perfectionism interferes with treatment progress?" and "What strategies do you use to help perfectionistic clients tolerate making mistakes in therapy?" Understanding their perfectionism approach is crucial for quiet BPD treatment.

Ask about family and relationship involvement: "Do you involve family members or partners in treatment for quiet BPD clients?" and "How do you address relationship patterns that maintain quiet BPD symptoms?" These questions help determine their understanding of the interpersonal aspects of quiet BPD.

Insurance navigation guide

Understanding insurance coverage for mental health treatment helps you access appropriate care while managing costs effectively. Insurance navigation for quiet BPD treatment requires understanding both general mental health benefits and specific considerations for personality disorder treatment.

Understanding Your Mental Health Benefits

Coverage basics for mental health treatment are governed by mental health parity laws that require insurance companies to provide mental health benefits comparable to medical benefits. Your insurance plan should cover therapy sessions, psychiatric evaluations, and other mental health services at similar rates to medical care.

Review your **Summary of Benefits** document to understand your mental health coverage specifics. Look for information about therapy session copays, annual deductibles that apply to mental health services, out-of-network coverage percentages and requirements, and any limits on the number of therapy sessions per year.

In-network versus out-of-network providers significantly affects your costs and coverage. In-network therapists have contracted rates with your insurance company and typically require lower copays, while out-of-network providers may require you to pay full fees upfront and seek reimbursement, often with higher deductibles and lower reimbursement percentages.

Personality Disorder Coverage Considerations

Some insurance plans have **specific limitations** for personality disorder treatment that don't apply to other mental health conditions. Review your plan documents for any exclusions or limitations related to personality disorders, requirements for preauthorization for personality disorder treatment, limits on session frequency or treatment duration for personality disorders, and specific requirements for treatment provider qualifications.

Documentation requirements for personality disorder treatment may be more stringent than for other conditions. Your therapist may need to provide detailed treatment plans and progress reports, justify the medical necessity of continued treatment, and document specific symptoms and functional impairments to maintain coverage approval.

Diagnostic coding affects coverage, and some therapists may initially use anxiety or depression codes rather than personality disorder codes to ensure coverage approval. While this practice is common, discuss with your therapist how diagnostic coding might affect your treatment planning and insurance coverage over time.

Maximizing Your Benefits

Flexible Spending Accounts (FSA) or **Health Savings Accounts (HSA)** can help manage mental health treatment costs. These accounts allow you to pay for qualified mental health expenses with pre-tax dollars, including therapy copays, psychiatric medications, and some mental health-related materials and programs.

Employee Assistance Programs (EAP) often provide free short-term counseling services that can supplement your regular therapy. While EAP counselors may not specialize in quiet BPD, they can provide additional support during difficult periods and help you navigate other life stresses that affect your mental health.

Coverage appeals may be necessary if your insurance company denies coverage for treatments your therapist recommends. The appeals process typically involves your therapist providing additional documentation about the medical necessity of treatment, you submitting a formal written appeal within specified timeframes, and potentially participating in peer review processes where other mental health professionals evaluate your case.

Low-cost therapy options

Accessing quality mental health care when cost is a concern requires exploring various alternative options and funding sources. Many communities offer reduced-cost services that can provide appropriate treatment for quiet BPD presentations.

Community Mental Health Centers

Federally Qualified Health Centers (FQHCs) provide mental health services on a sliding fee scale based on your income and family size. These centers are required to serve patients regardless of insurance status or ability to pay, and many employ therapists trained in evidence-based treatments including those appropriate for personality disorders.

Community mental health organizations often provide specialized services for various mental health conditions, including personality disorders. These organizations may offer individual therapy, group therapy, psychiatric services, and case management at reduced rates based on financial need.

University training clinics provide therapy services delivered by graduate students under professional supervision. While students are still learning, they often have access to current research and evidence-based treatments, and their services are typically offered at significantly reduced rates. Many university clinics have specific programs for personality disorder treatment.

Faith-Based and Nonprofit Organizations

Religious organizations often provide counseling services through trained pastoral counselors or licensed therapists who work within faith communities. These services may be free or low-cost and can be appropriate even if you don't share the organization's religious beliefs, though it's important to discuss this upfront.

Nonprofit mental health organizations focus on providing accessible mental health services to underserved populations. These organizations may offer sliding scale fees, scholarships for treatment costs, specialized programs for specific populations or conditions, and connections to other community resources and support services.

Peer support organizations provide services delivered by people with lived experience of mental health conditions. While peer support doesn't replace professional therapy, it can provide valuable supplemental support at low or no cost and help you develop coping skills and community connections.

Alternative Funding and Support Options

Treatment scholarships and grants are sometimes available through mental health organizations, professional associations, or private foundations. These funding sources may provide full or partial coverage for therapy costs, particularly for individuals with limited financial resources or specific demographic characteristics.

Therapy training programs sometimes offer reduced-cost services as part of therapist certification or continuing education requirements. Licensed therapists working toward specialized certifications may provide services at reduced rates while receiving supervision in specific treatment modalities.

Online therapy platforms increasingly offer sliding scale pricing or financial assistance programs. While online therapy isn't appropriate for all situations, it can provide access to qualified therapists at lower costs than traditional in-person services, particularly for ongoing maintenance therapy or skill-building support.

International resources directory

Access to appropriate mental health care varies significantly across different countries and healthcare systems. This directory provides starting points for finding quiet BPD treatment and support in various international locations.

English-Speaking Countries

United Kingdom provides mental health services through the National Health Service (NHS), though wait times for specialized personality disorder treatment can be extensive. Private therapy options include British Association for Counselling and Psychotherapy (BACP) member therapists, Priory Group facilities that specialize in personality disorders, and online therapy platforms available in the UK.

Specific resources include NHS Improving Access to Psychological Therapies (IAPT) services for initial assessment and treatment, Mind UK for mental health information and local support groups, and Rethink Mental Illness for specialized personality disorder resources and advocacy.

Canada offers mental health services through provincial healthcare systems, with coverage varying by province. Resources include Canadian Psychological Association (CPA) therapist directories, Centre for Addiction and Mental Health (CAMH) in Ontario for specialized treatment, and provincial mental health organizations that provide information and support services.

Australia provides mental health services through Medicare with subsidized therapy sessions. Resources include Australian Psychological Society (APS) therapist directories, Beyond Blue for mental health information and support, and state-based mental health organizations that offer specialized services and support groups.

European Countries

Germany offers mental health services through statutory health insurance with coverage for therapy and psychiatric treatment. Resources include German Society for Psychology (DGPs) therapist directories, federal and state mental health information centers, and specialized clinics that provide personality disorder treatment.

Netherlands provides mental health care through mandatory health insurance that covers therapy and psychiatric treatment. Resources include Netherlands Institute of Psychologists (NIP) therapist directories, GGZ Nederland mental health organizations, and specialized personality disorder treatment centers.

France offers mental health services through the national healthcare system with coverage for therapy and psychiatric care. Resources include French Federation of Psychologists (FFP) therapist directories, regional mental health centers (CMP), and specialized hospital departments that provide personality disorder treatment.

Asian Countries

Japan has increasing mental health awareness though cultural stigma remains significant. Resources include Japanese Association of Clinical Psychology therapist directories, national and prefectural mental health centers, and online resources available in both Japanese and English for expatriate communities.

Singapore provides mental health services through public healthcare with some private options. Resources include Singapore Psychological Society therapist directories, Institute of Mental Health (IMH) for specialized treatment, and expatriate community mental health resources.

South Korea offers mental health services through national health insurance with growing awareness of personality disorders. Resources include Korean Psychological Association therapist directories, specialized university hospital departments, and international clinic services for English-speaking patients.

Support for International Communities

Expatriate mental health resources are available in many countries through international clinics, expatriate community organizations, embassy or consulate mental health information, and online therapy platforms that serve international populations.

Teletherapy across borders is increasingly available though legal and licensing requirements vary. Some therapists are licensed to provide services internationally, online platforms may offer services to expatriates, and some organizations specialize in providing therapy to specific international communities.

Language and cultural considerations affect treatment access and effectiveness. Look for therapists who speak your native language fluently, understand your cultural background and values, have experience working with expatriate or immigrant populations, and can provide culturally adapted treatment approaches when appropriate.

Appendix D: Quick reference guides

DBT skills cheat sheet for quiet BPD

Traditional DBT skills require adaptation for quiet BPD presentations because the standard approaches assume you need to decrease emotional intensity rather than increase emotional awareness and expression. This cheat sheet provides modified DBT techniques specifically designed for internalized presentations.

Mindfulness Skills for Quiet BPD

Observe your internal landscape rather than external events when practicing mindfulness. Standard DBT mindfulness often focuses on environmental awareness, but quiet BPD requires attention to subtle internal states. Practice noticing physical sensations that indicate suppressed emotions, thoughts that minimize or dismiss your experiences, urges to suppress or avoid emotional content, and moments when you disconnect from your authentic feelings.

Describe emotions with precision and validation instead of minimizing their significance. Quiet BPD often involves sophisticated emotional suppression that requires intentional counteraction. When describing your emotional experience, use specific emotion words rather than general terms like "fine" or "stressed," acknowledge the full intensity of your emotions even when others can't see them, validate your emotional responses as understandable given your circumstances, and avoid immediately jumping to problem-solving mode when experiencing difficult emotions.

Participate authentically in activities rather than going through the motions while emotionally disconnected. Quiet BPD often involves mechanistic participation in life activities without genuine engagement. Practice choosing activities based on your authentic preferences rather than others' expectations, allowing yourself to experience genuine enjoyment or displeasure with activities, expressing your authentic reactions to experiences rather than expected responses, and engaging fully with chosen activities rather than multitasking or mental distraction.

Emotion Regulation Skills Adaptations

Increase emotional awareness before attempting regulation strategies. Traditional DBT assumes you can identify your emotions, but quiet BPD often requires foundational work in emotional recognition. Practice regular body scans to identify physical manifestations of emotions, emotion naming exercises using detailed feeling words, tracking emotional patterns over time to identify subtle variations, and connecting emotions to their underlying needs or values.

Express emotions appropriately rather than suppressing them entirely. Standard emotion regulation often focuses on reducing emotional expression, but quiet BPD requires learning healthy expression. Practice sharing emotions in low-risk situations to build comfort, expressing needs and preferences clearly and directly, using "I" statements to communicate emotional experiences, and setting appropriate boundaries around emotional expression without complete suppression.

Challenge emotion myths that maintain emotional suppression patterns. Quiet BPD often involves beliefs that emotions are inappropriate, burdensome, or dangerous. Work on recognizing thoughts like "others have it worse, so I shouldn't feel this way," "expressing emotions is selfish and burdens others," "strong people handle things without getting emotional," and "if I start crying, I'll never stop."

Interpersonal Effectiveness Adaptations

Ask for what you need without excessive self-justification or minimization. Traditional interpersonal effectiveness assumes basic comfort with making requests, but quiet BPD often involves severe difficulty with need expression. Practice identifying your needs and wants before interpersonal situations, making direct requests without extensive apologies or justifications, accepting that others may decline your requests without catastrophizing, and distinguishing between wants and needs to prioritize appropriately.

Express disagreement respectfully while maintaining your authentic position. Quiet BPD often involves suppressing disagreement to avoid conflict, which requires specific skill development. Practice expressing different opinions in low-stakes situations, using phrases like "I see it differently" or "My experience has been different," staying focused on specific behaviors or situations rather than character judgments, and maintaining respect for others while honoring your own perspective.

Set boundaries without excessive guilt by focusing on your legitimate needs and limits. Boundary setting often triggers intense guilt and fear in quiet BPD presentations. Practice saying no to requests that exceed your capacity or conflict with your values, explaining your limits clearly without over-justification, tolerating others' disappointment without changing your boundaries, and distinguishing between reasonable accommodation and self-abandonment.

Distress Tolerance Modifications

Tolerate emotional intensity rather than immediately suppressing difficult feelings. Standard distress tolerance focuses on surviving emotional crises, but quiet BPD requires learning to stay present with emotions that feel uncomfortable but aren't actually dangerous. Practice sitting with emotions for short periods without attempting to change them, using breathing techniques to stay grounded during emotional experiences, reminding yourself that emotions are temporary and will naturally decrease over time, and seeking appropriate support during difficult emotional periods.

Use crisis survival skills for internal emotional emergencies rather than external behavioral crises. Quiet BPD crises often involve internal emotional states that feel unbearable but aren't visible to others. Adapt traditional crisis skills by creating safe physical environments when feeling emotionally overwhelmed, using intensive self-soothing techniques during periods of emotional numbness or despair, reaching out for support even when you feel like you're being a burden, and maintaining basic self-care during difficult periods even when motivation is low.

Communication scripts for difficult conversations

People with quiet BPD often struggle with initiating difficult conversations because they fear conflict, worry about being a burden, or lack experience with direct communication. These scripts provide starting points for various challenging situations while allowing for your personal style and specific circumstances.

Setting Boundaries Scripts

Declining requests politely but firmly: "I appreciate you thinking of me for this opportunity, but I won't be able to take this on right now. I hope you find someone who can give it the attention it deserves." This script acknowledges the request positively while providing a clear decline without extensive justification.

Setting limits with persistent requests: "I understand this is important to you, and I've given it careful consideration. My answer remains no, and I'd appreciate it if we don't revisit this topic again." This script maintains respect while clearly establishing that the boundary isn't open for renegotiation.

Expressing capacity limits: "I care about you and want to support you, but I'm not in a good place to provide the kind of help you need right now. Have you considered talking to [specific alternative resource]?" This script shows care while clearly stating your limits and offering alternative support.

Addressing overcommitment patterns: "I realize I've been taking on more than I can handle effectively. I need to step back from some commitments to maintain the quality of work I want to provide. I'll be reducing my involvement in [specific activities] starting [timeframe]."

This script takes responsibility while clearly stating changes you need to make.

Expressing Needs and Preferences

Requesting support directly: "I'm going through a difficult time right now and could use some support. Would you be willing to [specific request] sometime in the next week? It would really help me manage things better." This script is direct about your need while making a specific, time-limited request.

Expressing preferences in group settings: "I have a different preference on this. I'd like us to consider [alternative option] because [brief reason]. How does that sound to everyone else?" This script expresses your view while inviting others' input and maintaining collaborative tone.

Asking for accommodations: "I have some needs that would help me participate more effectively. Would it be possible to [specific accommodation]? This would allow me to contribute more fully to our work together." This script frames accommodations as ways to enhance your contribution rather than special treatment.

Requesting changes in established patterns: "I've been thinking about our [routine/arrangement], and I'd like to suggest some changes that would work better for me. Could we talk about adjusting [specific aspect] to [proposed change]?" This script introduces change requests as discussion topics rather than demands.

Addressing Relationship Issues

Expressing relationship concerns: "I've been feeling some distance in our relationship lately, and I'd like to talk about it. I'm wondering if you've noticed anything different, and I'd love to hear your thoughts about how we can reconnect." This script opens dialogue without blame while expressing your observations.

Requesting more emotional intimacy: "I really value our relationship, and I'd love for us to share more about what's happening in our lives. I sometimes feel like we stick to surface-level topics, and I'm interested in deeper conversations. How would you feel about that?" This script expresses your desire for deeper connection while checking the other person's comfort level.

Addressing recurring conflicts: "I've noticed we keep having similar conversations about [issue], and I'm wondering if we can approach this differently. What do you think is underneath this pattern, and how can we address the core issue?" This script moves beyond specific incidents to address underlying patterns.

Discussing mental health with loved ones: "I want to share something with you that's been affecting me. I've been working with a therapist on some emotional patterns, and part of that involves being more open about my experiences. I'd appreciate your support as I work on being more authentic in our relationship." This script introduces your mental health work as something that will enhance your relationship.

Workplace accommodation request templates

Requesting workplace accommodations for mental health conditions requires balancing legal rights with practical considerations and workplace relationships. These templates provide structures for various accommodation requests while maintaining professional presentation.

General Accommodation Request Framework

Initial accommodation request: "I am writing to request workplace accommodations under the Americans with Disabilities Act due to a medical condition that affects my work performance. I am able to perform the essential functions of my job with reasonable accommodations. I would like to schedule a meeting to discuss specific accommodations that would help me maintain my productivity and effectiveness."

Medical documentation statement: "I am providing documentation from my healthcare provider confirming that I have a qualifying condition and outlining recommended workplace accommodations. I am committed to working with you to implement accommodations that meet both my needs and the company's operational requirements."

Confidentiality request: "I request that information about my condition and accommodations be kept confidential and shared only with individuals who need this information to implement the accommodations or as required by law. I appreciate your commitment to maintaining my privacy while ensuring I receive appropriate support."

Specific Accommodation Templates

Flexible schedule request: "I am requesting a flexible work schedule as an accommodation for my medical condition. Specifically, I would like to [adjust start/end times, work from home certain days, have flexibility for medical appointments]. This accommodation would allow me to manage my condition effectively while maintaining full productivity in my role."

Workload modification request: "I am requesting modifications to my workload structure as a reasonable accommodation. This could include [prioritizing essential tasks during difficult periods, extending deadlines when needed, redistributing non-essential responsibilities]. I remain committed to meeting all essential job requirements with these adjustments."

Communication accommodation request: "I am requesting accommodations related to communication and feedback processes. Specifically, I would benefit from [written instructions for complex tasks, regular check-ins to ensure understanding, advance notice of major changes when possible]. These accommodations would help me perform more effectively and reduce workplace stress."

Break and leave accommodation request: "I am requesting additional break time and flexible leave options as accommodations for my medical condition. This might include [additional short breaks during the day, flexibility to take mental health days, ability to step away briefly when experiencing symptoms]. I will coordinate with my supervisor to ensure coverage and minimal disruption."

Follow-Up and Maintenance Templates

Accommodation effectiveness review: "I wanted to provide an update on how the current accommodations are working and discuss any needed adjustments. [Specific accommodation] has been very helpful in allowing me to maintain productivity. I would like to discuss [any needed modifications] to ensure continued effectiveness."

New accommodation request: "As my role has evolved, I would like to request additional accommodations that would help me continue performing effectively. Specifically, I am requesting [new accommodation] because [brief explanation of need]. I believe this would enhance my ability to contribute to our team's success."

Accommodation renewal: "My current accommodations are scheduled for review, and I would like to request their continuation. These accommodations continue to be necessary for me to perform my job effectively, and I am grateful for the company's support in providing them. I am happy to provide updated medical documentation if needed."

Family psychoeducation summary

Family members and loved ones need concise, accurate information about quiet BPD to provide appropriate support while maintaining their own wellbeing. This summary provides essential information for family members who want to understand and support their loved one's recovery journey.

Understanding Quiet BPD Basics

What quiet BPD looks like: Your loved one experiences the same emotional intensity and relationship difficulties as people with traditional BPD, but they direct these struggles inward rather than expressing them externally. They may appear successful, controlled, and emotionally stable while privately experiencing overwhelming emotions, self-criticism, and fear of abandonment.

How it differs from traditional BPD: Instead of dramatic outbursts or obvious behavioral problems, people with quiet BPD typically suppress their emotions, avoid conflict, maintain perfect appearances, and experience intense internal distress that others rarely see. Their symptoms are designed to be invisible, which often leads to delayed diagnosis and treatment.

Why external success doesn't indicate wellbeing: Professional achievements, social functioning, and maintained responsibilities don't negate the reality of internal emotional struggles. Your loved one may work harder to maintain external success precisely because they fear that any imperfection will result in rejection or abandonment.

Common symptoms you might notice: Changes in sleep patterns, appetite, or energy levels; subtle withdrawal from emotional intimacy; increased perfectionism or people-pleasing behaviors; physical complaints without clear medical causes; and difficulty making decisions or expressing preferences.

How to Provide Helpful Support

Validation approaches that help: Acknowledge their emotional experiences without trying to fix them immediately, express appreciation for their willingness to share struggles with you, recognize the strength it takes to seek help and work on personal growth, and avoid minimizing their struggles because their external life appears successful.

Communication strategies: Ask open-ended questions about their experiences rather than making assumptions, listen without immediately offering advice or solutions, express your observations about changes you've noticed without making accusations, and check in regularly about their wellbeing without being intrusive.

Boundaries that support recovery: Maintain your own emotional wellbeing and activities rather than focusing exclusively on their struggles, avoid taking responsibility for their treatment decisions or emotional reactions, offer specific types of support rather than unlimited availability, and encourage their independence and decision-making capabilities.

What not to do: Don't tell them they should be grateful because their life looks good from the outside, don't suggest they just need to think more positively or try harder, don't take on their responsibilities to prevent them from experiencing natural consequences, and don't violate their privacy by sharing their struggles with others without permission.

Supporting Treatment and Recovery

Understanding the treatment process: Recovery from quiet BPD typically takes time and involves gradual changes rather than dramatic transformations, setbacks are normal parts of the process rather than signs of treatment failure, and progress might be subtle and difficult to recognize without looking for specific changes.

How to support their treatment: Respect their privacy while expressing interest in their progress, avoid pressuring them to share details about therapy sessions, support their treatment decisions even when you don't fully understand them, and be patient with the pace of change while maintaining hope for continued improvement.

Recognizing positive changes: Increased willingness to express needs or preferences, greater comfort with making mistakes or receiving criticism, improved ability to set boundaries or say no to requests, more authentic emotional expression, and decreased anxiety about others' opinions or reactions.

Crisis support guidelines: Take seriously any expressions of suicidal thoughts or self-harm urges, help them access professional crisis support when needed, maintain consistent caring contact without becoming responsible for their safety, and know the warning signs that indicate they need immediate professional intervention.

Maintaining Your Own Wellbeing

Self-care essentials: Continue your own interests, activities, and relationships rather than focusing exclusively on your loved one's struggles, seek your own support through friends, family, or your own therapy when needed, and maintain realistic expectations about your ability to help or influence their recovery process.

Understanding your limits: You cannot cure or control their condition through love and support alone, their progress or setbacks don't reflect your adequacy as a family member or friend, and providing good support sometimes means saying no to requests that exceed your capacity.

Resources for family members: Consider family therapy or support groups for relatives of people with personality disorders, educate yourself about quiet BPD through reliable resources, and maintain connections with other supportive people in your life rather than isolating yourself.

Building a supportive family environment: Focus on authentic connection rather than perfect harmony, model healthy emotional expression and boundary-setting, celebrate small improvements and progress rather than waiting for dramatic changes, and create family traditions and interactions that emphasize genuine connection over performance or achievement.

These reference guides provide practical tools for navigating the ongoing challenges and opportunities that arise in quiet BPD recovery. Keep them accessible for moments when you need quick guidance or reminders about healthy approaches to common situations.

The journey of understanding and healing from quiet BPD involves learning new ways of relating to yourself and others that honor both your emotional depth and your need for authentic connection. These tools support that journey by providing concrete strategies and frameworks for the challenges you'll encounter along the way.

Key Takeaways for Using These Resources:

- Assessment tools help track progress and identify patterns that might not be obvious day-to-day
- Continued learning resources support your ongoing growth and understanding of quiet BPD
- Finding appropriate professional help requires asking specific questions about experience and approach
- Communication scripts provide starting points that you can adapt to your personal style and specific situations
- Workplace accommodations are legal rights that can help you maintain professional success while managing your condition
- Family psychoeducation helps loved ones provide appropriate support while maintaining their own wellbeing

References

- Betts, J., Chanen, A., Crowley, R., Frøland, A., Grenyer, B. F. S., Laurenssen, E., McCutcheon, L., ... & Sharp, C. (2018). A psychoeducational group intervention for family and friends of youth with borderline personality disorder features: Protocol for a randomized controlled trial. *Borderline Personality Disorder and Emotion Dysregulation, 5*, 16. https://doi.org/10.1186/s40479-018-0090-z

- Brunner, R., Henze, R., Parzer, P., Kramer, J., Feigl, N., Lutz, K., Essig, M., & Resch, F. (2014). Reduced cortical and subcortical volumes in female adolescents with borderline personality disorder. *Psychiatry Research: Neuroimaging, 221*(3), 179–186. https://doi.org/10.1016/j.pscychresns.2012.07.002

- Choosing Therapy. (2023). Quiet borderline personality disorder: Signs, symptoms, & treatments. https://www.choosingtherapy.com/quiet-borderline-personality-disorder/

- Degasperi, G., Minichino, A., Maffei, C., & Brambilla, P. (2021). Parsing variability in borderline personality disorder: A meta-analysis of neuroimaging studies. *Translational Psychiatry, 11*, 314. https://doi.org/10.1038/s41398-021-01446-z

- Ding, J. B., & Hu, K. (2021). Structural MRI brain alterations in borderline personality disorder and bipolar disorder. *Cureus, 13*(7), e16425. https://doi.org/10.7759/cureus.16425

- Eggshell Therapy. (2022). Quiet borderline personality disorder: Suffering in silence. https://eggshelltherapy.com/quiet-bpd/

- Grouport Therapy. (2019). The quiet episode in borderline personality disorder: Understanding and coping strategies. https://www.grouporttherapy.com/blog/quiet-episode-bpd

- Guillén, V., Marco, J. H., Gracia, R., Perpiñá, C., Baños, R. M., Botella, C., & Espada, J. P. (2022). Effectiveness of the "Family Connections" program versus treatment-as-usual for relatives of individuals with borderline personality disorder: A randomized controlled trial. *Journal of Clinical Psychology, 78*(7), 1361–1376. https://doi.org/10.1002/jclp.23296

- Healthline. (2022). Quiet borderline personality disorder: Symptoms, causes, diagnosis, & treatment. https://www.healthline.com/health/quiet-bpd

- Heal Treatment Centers. (2022). Quiet borderline personality disorder explained clearly. https://healtreatmentcenters.com/mental-health/quiet-borderline-personality-disorder/

- Iskric, A., & Barkley-Levenson, E. (2021). Neural changes in borderline personality disorder after dialectical behavior therapy: A review. *Frontiers in Psychiatry, 12,* 772081. https://doi.org/10.3389/fpsyt.2021.772081

- Laurini, O., Strugarek, P., & Rahioui, H. (2025). Borderline personality: Revisiting its classification as a neurodevelopmental disorder. *Frontiers in Psychiatry, 16,* 1587778. https://doi.org/10.3389/fpsyt.2025.1587778

- Leichsenring, F., Fonagy, P., Heim, N., Kernberg, O. F., Leweke, F., Luyten, P., Salzer, S., Spitzer, C., & Steinert, C. (2024). Borderline personality disorder: A comprehensive review of diagnosis and clinical presentation, etiology, treatment, and current controversies. *World Psychiatry, 23*(1), 4–25. https://doi.org/10.1002/wps.21156

- López-Villatoro, J. M., Díaz-Marsá, M., Mellor-Marsá, B., De la Vega, I., & Carrasco, J. L. (2020). Executive dysfunction associated with the primary psychopathic features of borderline personality disorder. *Frontiers in Psychiatry, 11,* 514905. https://doi.org/10.3389/fpsyt.2020.514905

- May, J. M., Richardi, T. M., & Barth, K. S. (2016). Dialectical behavior therapy as treatment for borderline personality disorder. *Mental Health Clinician, 6*(2), 62–67. https://doi.org/10.9740/mhc.2016.03.62

- Modern Intimacy. (2021). 8 ways to identify quiet borderline personality disorder. https://www.modernintimacy.com/8-ways-to-identify-quiet-borderline-personality-disorder/

- My Psychiatrist. (2022). What is quiet borderline personality disorder (BPD)? https://mypsychiatrist.com/blog/what-is-quiet-bpd/

- NAMI (National Alliance on Mental Illness). (2022). Borderline personality disorder. https://www.nami.org/about-mental-illness/mental-health-conditions/borderline-personality-disorder/

- National Collaborating Centre for Mental Health (UK). (2009). *Borderline personality disorder: Treatment and management* (NICE Clinical Guideline CG78). British Psychological Society & Royal College of Psychiatrists. https://www.ncbi.nlm.nih.gov/books/NBK55407/

- Pearce, J., Knight, T., & Hiskey, S. (2017). Evaluation of the "Making Sense of BPD" psychoeducational group intervention for family and friends of youth with borderline personality disorder: A pilot study. *Borderline Personality Disorder and Emotion Dysregulation, 4*, 9. https://doi.org/10.1186/s40479-017-0056-6

- Pitschel-Walz, G., Spatzl, A., & Rentrop, M. (2022). Psychoeducational groups for close relatives of patients with borderline personality disorder. *European Archives of Psychiatry and Clinical Neuroscience, 273*(1), 113–122. https://doi.org/10.1007/s00406-022-01395-8

- Priory Group. (2021). What is quiet BPD? Signs, traits and support. https://www.priorygroup.com/blog/quiet-borderline-personality-disorder

- Psych Central. (2021). What is "quiet" borderline personality disorder? Symptoms, treatment & resources. https://psychcentral.com/disorders/borderline-personality-disorder/quiet-bpd

- Psychology Today. (2019). Do you have "quiet" borderline personality disorder? *Living with Emotional Intensity.* https://www.psychologytoday.com/us/blog/living-with-emotional-intensity/201909/do-you-have-quiet-bpd

- Rethink Mental Illness. (2023). Living with borderline personality disorder: Rachel's story. https://www.rethink.org/news-and-stories/blogs/2023/07/living-with-borderline-personality-disorder-rachels-story/

- Schulze, L., Schmahl, C., & Niedtfeld, I. (2016). Neural correlates of disturbed emotion processing in borderline personality disorder: A multimodal meta-analysis. *Biological Psychiatry, 79*(2), 97–106. https://doi.org/10.1016/j.biopsych.2015.03.027

- StatPearls Publishing. (2024). Borderline personality disorder. In *StatPearls* [Internet]. StatPearls Publishing. https://www.ncbi.nlm.nih.gov/books/NBK430883/

- Steele, K. R., Townsend, M. L., & Grenyer, B. F. S. (2020). Parenting stress and competence in borderline personality disorder is associated with mental health, trauma history, attachment and reflective capacity. *Borderline Personality Disorder and Emotion Dysregulation, 7*, 8. https://doi.org/10.1186/s40479-020-00124-8

- Whittle, S., Chanen, A. M., Fornito, A., McGorry, P. D., Pantelis, C., & Yücel, M. (2009). Anterior cingulate volume in adolescents with first-presentation borderline personality disorder. *Psychiatry Research: Neuroimaging, 172*(2), 155–160. https://doi.org/10.1016/j.pscychresns.2008.12.004